start right baby a

essentials

catherine atkinson

foulsham
LONDON • NEW YORK • TORONTO • SYDNEY

foulsham
The Publishing House, Bennetts Close,
Cippenham, Berks, SL1 5AP, England

ISBN 0-572-02974-8

Copyright © 2004 W. Foulsham & Co. Ltd

A CIP record for this book is available from the British Library

Front cover photograph reproduced with kind permission from The Image Bank

All rights reserved.

The Copyright Act prohibits (subject to certain very limited exceptions) the making of copies of any copyright work or of a substantial part of such a work, including the making of copies by photocopying or similar process. Written permission to make a copy or copies must therefore normally be obtained from the publisher in advance. It is advisable to consult the publisher if in any doubt as to the legality of any copying which is to be undertaken.

Neither the editors of W. Foulsham & Co. Ltd nor the author nor the publisher takes responsibility for any possible consequences from any action by any person reading or following the information in this book.

Printed in Great Britain by Cox & Wyman Ltd, Reading

Contents

Introduction	4
The Best Food for Your Baby	6
Notes on the Recipes	24
About Four Months	25
About Five Months	35
Six to Nine Months	56
Nine to Twelve Months	93
From Baby to Toddler	132
Index	186

Introduction

Weaning is the gradual process of introducing solid food to a baby who has relied entirely on breast or formula milk. It's an important and rewarding stage in your baby's development, but can also be a frustrating and confusing time: when it comes to feeding babies, the world seems to be full of people giving conflicting advice on what, when and how!

In this book you'll find plenty of help to guide you through the next 12 months or so, from those first few spoonfuls to the point when your child will be joining in family meals. Your baby's progress will be gradual, starting with baby rice with a consistency only slightly thicker than milk, moving on to thin, smooth purées. As your baby grows, you will find you no longer need to purée the food and can mash it with a fork, then later simply chop it into small pieces. The chapters reflect this and are divided into the different stages of weaning, so you can take it step by step. Most of the recipes are quick and simple to prepare and can be made in larger quantities so that several portions can be frozen for future use.

Cooking for a baby can be fun, as well as being a healthier and cost-effective alternative to bland, processed meals from jars or packets. By serving a wide range of fresh, home-made food, you can help develop your baby's tastebuds to appreciate a variety of foods, flavours and textures throughout childhood and beyond. Remember that first impressions are lasting and that applies to first foods too!

Throughout the book you will find I have referred to the baby as 'she' – simply because all the recipes have been tried and tested over the years by my daughters, Harriet and Liz.

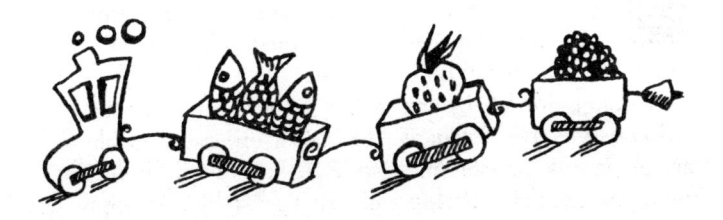

The Best Food for Your Baby

Babies have very different nutritional needs from adults. Their need for energy and protein is high in relation to their size during this stage of rapid growth and development. Forget about low-fat, high-fibre foods; they're great for adults but are not suitable for babies as they may fill up their stomachs before they can absorb all the nutrients they need.

Babies need as varied a diet as possible. Give your baby plenty of carbohydrate foods such as potatoes, rice, pasta, bread and cereals (but not the high-fibre varieties), vitamin-rich fruit and vegetables and a good helping of protein-rich foods such as meat, fish, eggs and dairy produce. Although fats and oils contain the essential fat-soluble vitamins A, D, E and K, don't add more than is necessary when preparing foods as your baby will get enough of these from foods such as meat and dairy produce. Most babies and children (and adults!) have a sweet tooth, but try to avoid sugary foods where possible, as these have little nutritional value, and never add salt to baby food as their kidneys are too immature to cope with it.

Although most babies are born with adequate stores of iron, these are used up by the age of about six months, so it's important to provide some iron-rich foods in the diet. Iron is found in concentrated amounts in meat and other foods, including egg yolks and, to a lesser extent, in pulses. Breakfast cereals and follow-on milk formula are also good sources as most are fortified with iron. Vitamin C helps the body to absorb iron, so offer vitamin-rich fruit and vegetables with or immediately after your baby's meals.

Vitamin drops are sometimes recommended for breast-fed babies and bottle-fed babies who are having less than 500 ml/ 17 fl oz/2¼ cups of milk formula daily. Ask your health visitor for advice on this.

Weaning from milk feeds to solids

During the first few months, breast or formula milk has provided all the nutrients babies need to grow and develop. But between four and six months they need more iron and other nutrients than can be provided by milk alone and may be ready to start on solids.

Signs that show your baby is ready for solids:

- ❖ Your baby still seems hungry after a milk feed and you've tried giving more milk.
- ❖ Your baby starts to demand feeds more frequently.
- ❖ Having started to sleep through the night, your baby starts waking again for a feed.
- ❖ Your baby seems interested in the food that you're eating and puts objects into her mouth to feel and chew.

Be guided by your own baby; if she's showing some or all of these signs, it's probably time to start giving solids. Babies progress at different rates and large babies occasionally need to start earlier than four months, though this is unusual. Check with your health visitor if you have any worries about when to start. Don't be pressurised by friends or relatives into starting sooner; you'll meet other parents who see weaning as a competition and believe that the sooner the better. Remember that a baby's digestive system is not fully matured in the first few months and that giving solids too early increases the chances of allergies later on. On the other hand, babies begin to learn how to chew at around six months, so don't delay starting solids after this age, or your baby may find it difficult to learn this skill.

Getting started

When you start giving your baby solid food you are simply introducing different tastes and textures and getting her used to feeding from a spoon. She still relies on her milk feeds for nourishment.

At first, offer food only once a day and introduce just one taste at a time. Baby rice cereal is an ideal first food as it's easy to digest. When mixed with breast or formula milk, the familiar taste and smell will help your baby relate to this new food. After a week or so, you can move on to fruit and mild-tasting vegetable purées. Apart from ripe bananas, these should always be cooked until very tender. At the beginning of weaning, food should have a very smooth, runny consistency, so you may need to thin purées with baby milk (breast or formula) or cooled, boiled water to achieve this.

When you introduce solids for the first time, choose a feed when your baby is alert and hungry but without being frantic; towards midday after a morning nap is usually a good choice. Give her a small milk feed to settle her and just take the edge off her hunger, then offer the solid food. Finish with the rest of the milk feed. Alternatively, you can try at the end of the milk feed if this works better.

At the beginning, the quantity of solids needed is minute – don't expect your baby to take more than a teaspoonful as her digestive system is still very immature. Remember, though, that you'll need to prepare at least double this amount as a lot of food will be dribbled straight back out rather than swallowed. Gradually build up the amount to 10–15 ml/2–3 tsp of food and when your baby happily takes one meal a day, you can move on to two meals a day.

Introducing solid food

Before starting to feed your baby, check that the food is at the right temperature. It should be just lukewarm; if it's too hot, you could put her off eating before she's tried her first spoonful! Next, protect your baby with a bib and have a damp flannel or kitchen paper (paper towels) to hand. Sit your baby upright in your lap, cradling her in your arm, so that she feels safe and secure. Later, when she's used to feeding, you may find it easier to feed her in a portable car seat or a bouncy baby chair on the floor. When she can sit up at about six or seven months, you can strap her into a highchair.

Weaning tips

- ❖ Scoop up a tiny amount of food on a small, plastic, sterilised spoon and gently place it between your baby's lips. Don't put the spoon in too far or she may gag.
- ❖ A lot of the food will probably be dribbled straight out again; it takes time to learn to feed from a spoon. Gently scrape it up and try again!
- ❖ If your baby doesn't like taking food from a spoon, try dipping a clean finger into the food and letting her suck the food off it.
- ❖ Go at your baby's pace, which will be slow. When she's had enough, she'll turn her head away.
- ❖ When your baby has finished, sit with her for a few minutes, keeping her in an upright position.
- ❖ If your baby is very reluctant to take solid foods and becomes upset, don't worry. Go back to breast or bottle feeding and try again in a few days' time.
- ❖ Never force your baby to take more food than she wants.

Buying equipment to get started

A visit to your local baby shop may make you think that you need masses of special equipment for weaning your baby. In fact you need very little, especially for the first few weeks, and you'll probably already have most of it in your kitchen.

The essentials

Plastic spoons You'll find spoons intended for weaning in baby-care shops and chemists. Babies can't lick food off a spoon at first, so these should be smooth with a shallow bowl that won't hurt your baby's gums.

Bibs Start with several fabric bibs with a plastic backing, the larger the better (puréed carrot goes a long way and stains badly!). When your baby sits up, you may prefer to use an easy-to-wash plastic 'pelican' bib with a trough to catch spills. Bibs with sleeves are also available for older babies who are starting to feed themselves.

Training beakers with a fitted lid and leakproof spout These are invaluable. A huge range is available: some have an interchangeable teat and spout, which is helpful when you want your baby to move on from a bottle to a drinking cup.

Plastic chopping boards These are better than wooden ones, which may harbour germs.

Fine plastic or stainless steel sieve (strainer) This is useful for removing pips and skins from puréed or mashed food.

Small heavy-based saucepan with a lid A small, good-quality pan is vital for cooking small quantities with minimal liquid.

Highchair When your baby is about six months old and her neck and back muscles can support her, a high chair will make feeding much easier. Shop around to find one that meets your needs. Many fold up to save space, others convert to a table and chair for when your baby becomes a toddler. Choose a model with a washable, non-fabric seat and tray; those with raised edges will catch any spills. Make sure that it is stable, with a secure safety harness, or hooks where one can be attached, to prevent your child climbing out. If you buy secondhand, check carefully for wear and tear. Where space (and money) is at a premium, you may prefer to opt for a clip-on chair that can be attached to a table or work surface. When your child is over 18 months, a booster seat strapped to an ordinary chair allow her to reach the table and will make her feel very grown-up!

The extras

Hand-held blender or liquidiser Although a fork or masher and a sieve (strainer) are perfectly adequate for making baby purées, an electric machine makes the job a lot quicker and easier, although you will still have to sieve some foods after puréeing to remove skins and pips. If you're buying new, choose one that can purée small quantities of food; family-sized blenders are designed to deal with large quantities and if you're only processing a small amount, the mixture tends to get stuck under the blades. A hand-turned food mill with fine and coarse cutting discs is a good alternative, as it purées the food and separates it from the skin and pips.

Steam steriliser or a cold solution Bottles and spoons can be sterilised in boiling water (see below), but a cold solution – where bottles and equipment are submerged in cold water and sterilising solution – or a steam steriliser is a good investment and easier to use.

Face cloths or baby wipes These are hygienic and handy for wiping sticky faces and hands (and other places where the food has reached!).

Plastic mat If you can't place the highchair on a floor that can be mopped clean, a mat is useful for catching any spills. Sheets of newspaper work just as well, with the added bonus that they can simply be rolled up afterwards and thrown away.

Food hygiene
Scares about food poisoning and media reports of salmonella and listeria cases have made parents especially aware of the importance of basic hygiene. Young babies pick up infections easily, but this can be prevented by following a few common-sense precautions when preparing food.

- ❖ Always wash your hands with hot water and soap before handling food or feeding equipment – an anti-bacterial handwash is ideal for this.
- ❖ It's important to continue sterilising bottles and teats until they are no longer used – warm milk is a wonderful

breeding ground for bacteria. You may feel that once your baby has started picking up things and putting them in her mouth it is pointless sterilising feeding equipment, but it's a good idea to sterilise feeding spoons and drinking beakers until your baby is a year old. This can be achieved by boiling in a saucepan of water for 25 minutes, by immersing in a container of cold water with sterilising fluid or tablets, or in a steam steriliser, following the manufacturer's instructions.

- ❖ It's impossible to sterilise all large equipment. Use a dishwasher if you have one, as it washes at a higher temperature than you can achieve by handwashing. Otherwise, wash feeding bowls, sieves (strainers), blenders, etc. by hand in soapy water, rinsing in clean hot water. Leave to air-dry in a rack, or use a clean tea towel (dish cloth) or kitchen paper (paper towels). Scald larger items such as chopping boards and knives with boiling water before using.
- ❖ Keep your work surfaces, chopping boards and utensils (choose plastic rather than wooden) scrupulously clean.
- ❖ If you have a pet, keep a separate can opener, fork and dish for its food and wash them up separately.
- ❖ Cool baby food as quickly as possible; putting the bowl or pan in a sink of iced water that comes about half way up the container will chill it quickly. Cover and refrigerate or freeze as soon as the food is cool.

Cooking and freezing baby food

Instead of cooking tiny amounts of food at each mealtime, prepare extra portions to freeze. Some foods don't freeze well, so if they are used in these recipes only chilling instructions are given. Never reheat more than once or refreeze thawed food.

To freeze puréed food, spoon into sterilised ice cube trays, open freeze until solid, then press the cubes out into plastic bags. Label the bags with the food and date and return to the freezer. Thaw the required number of cubes (one will be enough for a meal at first) and leave in a covered bowl at room temperature. Allow enough time for the food to defrost thoroughly. Heat until piping hot and allow to cool; always test before serving.

Larger portions must be thoroughly defrosted before reheating. This can be done at room temperature as long as the room is cool, but it is better to let them defrost in the fridge for at least 4 hours or overnight. Depending on the type of food, reheat in a saucepan on the hob, in the microwave on High, or in a covered dish in an oven preheated to 180°C/350°F/gas 4/fan oven 160°C. Test that the food is piping hot by inserting a thin knife or skewer into the centre for a few seconds; it should be very hot when removed. Then allow to cool before serving.

Freezer storage times (in a freezer at -18°C/0°F)

Purées containing milk	6 weeks
Meat, chicken and fish	2 months
Fruit and vegetables	4 months

The Best Food for Your Baby

Approximate ages for introducing new foods

Introduce new foods gradually so that your baby has a chance to get used to different tastes.

At four months
Baby rice
Cooked apple, papaya (pawpaw), pear
Ripe banana
Cooked carrots, courgette (zucchini), marrow (squash), parsnip, potato, squash, swede (rutabaga)

At five months
Non-wheat cereals, such as barley, oats, rye, soya
Kiwi fruit, melon, plums, raspberries
Spinach, celery, peas, leeks, sweetcorn (corn), cabbage, mushrooms, cauliflower, broccoli
Lentils and well-cooked pulses

At six months
Soaked dried fruit, such as apricots and peaches (but avoid raisins and sultanas (golden raisins))
Strawberries (see Allergies and food intolerance, page 21)
Tomatoes
Full-fat cows' milk in cooking
Dairy products, such as mild cheese, yoghurt, fromage frais
Tofu

White poultry meat, such as chicken and turkey
White fresh or frozen fish, such as cod, plaice and haddock
Cocoa (unsweetened chocolate) powder

At seven months
Pasta
Bread, breadsticks, crispbread, rusks
Citrus fruit
Fingers of cooked vegetables such as carrot
Cooked egg yolk
Lean red meat: beef and lamb

At nine months
Cooked whole eggs
Soaked raisins and sultanas (golden raisins)
Finely ground nuts (see Allergies and food intolerance, page 21)
Fresh or canned oily fish, such as sardines, mackerel, salmon and tuna
Sticks of raw fruit and vegetables

At one year
Shellfish (see Allergies and food intolerance, page 21)
Honey
Smooth peanut butter (see Allergies and food intolerance, page 21)

At three years
Whole nuts (see Allergies and food intolerance, page 21)

Milk matters

In the early stages of weaning, breast or formula milk will continue to provide most of the nutrients your baby needs and you should still be giving her at least 600 ml/1 pint/2½ cups a day, or four feeds if you are breastfeeding. As you continue with mixed feeding your baby will gradually demand fewer milk feeds, but milk will still be an important part of her diet.

By the age of six months, most babies are able to sip, rather than just suck, so start offering milk in a lidded feeder cup with meals at this time. You can breastfeed for as long as you want, but encourage your baby to give up the bottle by the age of one year, or the habit becomes very hard to break.

The UK Department of Health recommends that babies continue to have breast or formula milk throughout their first year. Follow-on milk formula can be introduced at six months and contains iron in a form that can be easily absorbed as well as vital vitamins. Cows' milk should not be given as a main drink before the age of one year because it contains only small amounts of iron and vitamin D and proteins that some babies find hard to digest. It can, however, be used in cooking from the age of six months.

Specially modified soya infant formulas are available for babies who have problems digesting breast or ordinary formula milk. They should only ever be given if advised by your doctor and you'll also need to speak to your dentist as their sugar content has been known to cause the developing teeth to decay.

When your child is about one year old, you can switch to full-fat (silver top) cows' milk. Aim to give a minimum of 350 ml/12 fl oz/1⅓ cups a day. For children who won't drink milk, give two servings of dairy products, such as cheese, fromage frais, yoghurt or milky desserts. After the age of two, you can swap to semi-skimmed milk if you prefer, provided your child is eating and growing satisfactorily. Skimmed milk is not suitable for children under five, as it is too low in calories and does not contain the fat-soluble vitamins A and D.

Other drinks

Always make sure that your baby has enough to drink, especially when the weather is hot. You can give water as well as milk. For babies under six months, tap water should always be boiled, then cooled. You can also give bottled water but this should also be boiled and cooled first. Do not give your baby carbonated, softened, those labelled 'natural mineral', or repeatedly boiled water because of the concentration of mineral salts it will contain.

At six months, you can start to introduce unsweetened fruit juice, such as apple or orange, diluting one part juice with three parts water and gradually increasing to half and half. These should be offered with, rather than between, meals as the fruit acids are harmful to the developing teeth. Some drinks manufactured specifically for babies and also many squashes contain surprising amounts of added sugar and should be avoided before the age of one. Check the label for sucrose, glucose, fructose, dextrose, maltose and honey – these are all forms of sugar.

Commercially prepared food

Although the emphasis of this book is that 'fresh is best', there are times when you'll find that pre-prepared jars, cans and packets of baby food are simply more convenient, especially when you're away from home. Dried baby foods are often useful during the early stages of weaning when you only need tiny amounts of food. Don't feel guilty about serving commercially prepared baby food when it suits you, but make sure your baby still gets variety and try to include plenty of fresh home-made food as well.

Vegetarian babies

A growing baby can get all the necessary nutrients from a diet excluding meat and fish, but it's important to balance the diet to ensure she gets enough protein, vitamins B12 and D, calcium and iron. Your baby can get plenty of protein from eggs, pulses, milk and dairy products including vegetarian cheese, tofu, finely ground nuts and nut spreads (see Allergies and food intolerance opposite). When she is over six months, puréed dried fruits, such as apricots and fortified breakfast cereals will provide iron in the diet. Vegetarian diets tend to be higher in fibre and therefore bulkier than those containing meat, so serve high-protein, low-fibre foods such as eggs and cheese daily.

If you choose to bring up your baby as a vegan and exclude all dairy foods and eggs from her diet, it is vitally important that you consult your doctor or health visitor, who should refer you to a dietician for specialist advice.

Whatever type of diet you decide on, have your baby weighed regularly at a health clinic; it'll reassure you that she's growing well and give you the chance to talk about any feeding problems you may have.

Allergies and food intolerance

Allergic reactions to food are extremely rare, but it's important to be aware of the symptoms, especially if there is a history of allergies in the family, as the results can be serious. The first noticeable reactions are usually red blotches on the skin and swelling of the face, eyes, mouth and tongue, often followed by nausea, vomiting and diarrhoea.

The allergen – the substance in the food that caused the reaction – may only produce very mild symptoms the first time the food is eaten, but if the child is repeatedly given the food, the symptoms will become increasingly severe. It's therefore important to introduce new foods one at a time and preferably at breakfast or lunchtime rather than last thing at night, so that you will immediately be aware of any problems should they

The Best Food for Your Baby

occur. If your child's mouth and tongue start to swell almost immediately after a trying a new food, seek medical help without delay.

Certain foods, like gluten which is found in wheat, are more likely to cause reactions. Others potential allergens are egg whites, nuts (especially peanuts), sesame seeds, shellfish, strawberries and cows' milk.

Food intolerance differs from an allergy and occurs when the digestive system doesn't produce the enzymes necessary to break down a certain food in the body. The most common is lactose intolerance – the inability to digest the sugars in milk due to an absence of the enzyme lactase. The enzyme may be absent at birth, or sometimes production of the enzyme stops after an illness such as gastroenteritis. If diagnosed, your doctor will advise you to switch to a soya milk formula. Some children who have an intolerance to lactose will still be able to eat dairy products such as yoghurt and cheese.

Making meal times easy

The meal planners in the subsequent chapters aim to help you through the early weeks and months of weaning but are intended as a guide only; there's no need to follow them rigidly – you can swap meals around or leave out certain ingredients as you wish. Don't feel that you have to prepare every meal for baby from scratch; save time and energy by making use of some of the vegetables you've cooked for the rest of the family – a few steamed carrots or a baked potato – but if you wish to add salt or strong spices to your food, remember to remove a portion for your baby first. Offering your baby home-made food will get her used to the food that the rest of the family eats, making things easier when it comes to joining in family meal times.

It's a good idea to serve the same food for two consecutive days, so that the baby can get used to each new flavour before introducing a new one – babies don't mind repetition, after all they've lived on milk alone for several months. If your baby rejects any new food with obvious dislike, go back to serving the foods she enjoys and try the new food again at a later date. Never make eating a battleground; just like adults, babies have likes and dislikes.

Notes on the Recipes

- All spoon measures are level: 1 tsp = 5 ml;
  1 tbsp = 15 ml.
- Ingredients are given in metric, imperial and American measures. Use only one set per recipe; do not interchange.
- Ensure that all produce is as fresh as possible.
- Always wash, peel, core and seed, if necessary, fresh fruit and vegetables before use.
- Avoid adding salt for babies or using ready-made products that are high in salt, such as some stock (bouillon) cubes, granules or powder.
- Use fresh herbs unless dried are specifically called for.
- All cooking times are approximate and are intended as a guide only.
- Always preheat the oven, unless it is a fan-assisted one, and cook on the centre shelf, unless otherwise stated.
- Recipes suitable for freezing are marked ✻.

About Four Months

These first mini-mouthfuls introduce your baby to a whole new experience in taste and texture. Make it a positive and happy time and she'll learn to see meal times as enjoyable occasions. Start by offering just a teaspoonful or two of baby rice mixed with baby milk (either breast or formula milk, whichever your baby is used to) to the consistency of single cream for the first week, then move on to runny fruit and vegetable purées. Gradually increase this to 10–15 ml/2–3 tsp at each meal and finally to two meals a day.

It isn't essential to start weaning your baby at exactly four months and you may decide to leave it a little longer, especially if there is a family history of allergies. See the advice on page 7 about when to start weaning and follow the pace that suits both you and your baby.

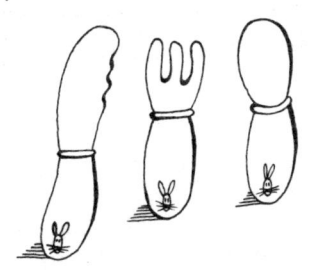

Foods to avoid at four months

- ❖ Citrus or soft berry fruits – these can cause allergic reactions in some babies.
- ❖ Cows' milk – give breast or formula milk instead.
- ❖ Eggs.
- ❖ Foods containing gluten, found in wheat including bread and some cereals, as your baby may find them difficult to digest.
- ❖ Meat, poultry, fish and shellfish.
- ❖ Nuts, including peanut butter and sesame seeds.
- ❖ Salt.
- ❖ Stock (bouillon) made from cubes, granules or powder.
- ❖ Sugar or honey – instead, choose naturally sweet, ripe fruit and mild-tasting vegetables such as young carrots and parsnips.

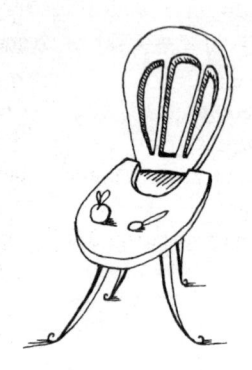

About Four Months

Four to five months meal planner

Week	Day	Lunch	Tea
1	Monday–Sunday	Baby rice (page 29)	
2	Monday	Banana purée (page 30)	
	Tuesday	Apple purée (page 30)	
	Wednesday	Apple purée (page 30)	
	Thursday	Carrot purée (page 33)	
	Friday	Carrot purée (page 33)	
	Saturday	Pear purée (page 31)	
	Sunday	Pear purée (page 31)	
3	Monday	Potato purée (page 34)	Banana purée (page 30)
	Tuesday	Banana purée (page 30)	Potato purée (page 34)
	Wednesday	Swede (rutabaga) purée (page 33)	Banana purée (page 30)
	Thursday	Cream of fruit purée (page 32)	Swede (rutabaga) purée (page 33)
	Friday	Butternut squash purée (page 34)	Cream of fruit purée (page 32)
	Saturday	Papaya (pawpaw) purée (page 31)	Butternut squash purée (page 34)
	Sunday	Parsnip purée (page 33)	Papaya (pawpaw) purée (page 31)

About Four Months

Week	Day	Lunch	Tea
4	Monday	Two-fruit purée (page 32)	Potato purée (page 34)
	Tuesday	Carrot purée (page 33)	Two-fruit purée (page 32)
	Wednesday	Apple purée (page 30)	Carrot purée (page 33)
	Thursday	Apple purée (page 30)	Parsnip purée (page 33)
	Friday	Pear purée (page 31)	Swede (rutabaga) purée (page 33)
	Saturday	Potato purée (page 34)	Pear purée (page 31)
	Sunday	Cream of fruit purée (page 32)	Potato purée (page 34)

Cooking purées in the microwave

Apple, pear and vegetable purées can be cooked in a microwave if preferred. Put the sliced or diced fruit or vegetable in a bowl with 15 ml/1 tbsp of water. Cover with clingfilm (plastic wrap), pierce in several places and cook on High for 5–6 minutes or until very tender. Purée, cool and serve as described in the individual recipes.

Baby rice

MAKES 1 BABY PORTION

Most baby rice cereals are fortified with vitamins and all should be salt- and sugar-free, but it's worth checking the packet to make sure. Spoon 10 ml/2 tsp of rice into a sterilised bowl. Stir in sufficient baby milk (breast or formula), according to the packet instructions, to make a smooth runny consistency. Check the temperature before feeding – it should be barely warm.

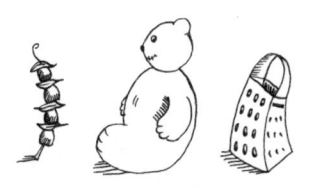

Banana purée

MAKES 1 BABY PORTION

Mash a 5 cm/2 in piece of very ripe banana with a fork to make it as smooth as possible, or press through a very fine sieve (strainer). Stir in 10–15 ml/2–3 tsp of baby milk (breast or formula) or cooled, boiled water to make a runny consistency. Serve straight away.

Apple purée

❋ **MAKES 4 BABY PORTIONS**

Peel, quarter and core 1 sweet eating (dessert) apple. Slice thinly and put in a small saucepan with 15 ml/1 tbsp of apple juice or water. Cover and simmer gently for 10 minutes or until very soft. Purée in a blender or press through a fine sieve (strainer). Spoon a quarter into a serving bowl and leave until tepid before serving. Cool the remainder and freeze in portions, or cover and store in the fridge for up to 24 hours.

Pear purée

❋ MAKES 4 BABY PORTIONS

Peel, quarter and core 1 ripe pear. Chop and put in a small saucepan with 15 ml/1 tbsp of water. Cover and simmer gently for 7–8 minutes or until very soft. Purée in a blender or press through a fine sieve (strainer). Spoon a quarter into a serving bowl and leave until tepid before serving. Cool the remainder and freeze in portions, or cover and store in the fridge for up to 24 hours.

Papaya purée

❋ MAKES 3 BABY PORTIONS

Thickly peel and remove the black seeds from ¼ ripe papaya (pawpaw). Put in a steamer or a sieve (strainer) placed over a pan of boiling water. Cover with a lid and steam for 3–4 minutes until very soft. Purée in a blender until smooth or press through a fine sieve. Spoon a third into a serving bowl and leave until tepid before serving. Cool the remainder and freeze in portions, or cover and store in the fridge for up to 24 hours.

Cream of fruit purée

MAKES 1 BABY PORTION

Mix 5 ml/1 tsp of baby rice with 10 ml/2 tsp of baby milk (breast or formula) or cooled, boiled water. Stir in 15 m/1 tbsp of apple, pear or papaya (pawpaw) purée (see pages 30 and 31).

Two-fruit purée

MAKES 1 BABY PORTION

Mash a 5 cm/2 in piece of very ripe banana with a fork until smooth or press through a very fine sieve (strainer). Stir in 15 ml/1 tbsp of apple, pear or papaya (pawpaw) purée (see pages 30 and 31) and a little cooled, boiled water, if needed, to make a runny consistency. Serve straight away.

Carrot, swede or parsnip purée

❊ MAKES 4 BABY PORTIONS

Trim and peel 100 g/4 oz of carrot, swede (rutabaga) or parsnip, then cut the vegetables into 2 cm/¾ in dice. Cook in a steamer or a sieve (strainer) placed over a pan of boiling water for 10–12 minutes until very soft. Purée in a blender or press though a fine sieve. Spoon a quarter into a serving bowl and leave to cool until tepid. Before serving, stir in enough baby milk (breast or formula) or cooled, boiled water to make the purée the desired consistency. Cool the remainder and freeze in portions, or cover and store in the fridge for up to 24 hours.

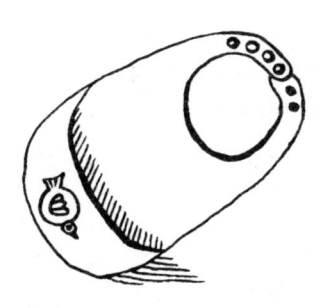

Potato purée

❇ MAKES 4 BABY PORTIONS

Wash a 100 g/4 oz potato and put it in a small saucepan. Barely cover the potato with boiling water and simmer for about 20 minutes until tender. Remove from the water and leave until it is cool enough to handle. Peel off the skin and mash until smooth. Add enough baby milk (breast or formula) to make the purée the desired consistency. Spoon a quarter into a serving bowl and leave until tepid before serving. Cool the remainder and freeze in portions, or cover and store in the fridge for up to 24 hours.

Alternatively, the potato can be baked in a preheated oven at 200°C/400°F/gas mark 6 for about 1 hour. Cut in half and scoop out the flesh. Mash as before.

Butternut squash purée

❇ MAKES 2 BABY PORTIONS

Peel and scoop out the seeds from 100 g/4 oz of butternut squash. Cut the flesh into 2.5 cm/1 in cubes and place in a steamer, or in a sieve (strainer) over a pan of boiling water. Cook for 7–8 minutes or until very tender. Purée in a blender or press through a fine sieve. Spoon half into a serving bowl and leave until tepid before serving. Cool the remainder and freeze, or cover and store in the fridge for up to 24 hours.

About Five Months

By now your baby should be taking (or soon will be) three small solid meals a day and is ready for a slightly more adventurous diet. She may now eat a wider variety of fruit and vegetables with the addition of poultry and fish. Food should still be puréed until smooth, but can be slightly thicker than before. New foods should be introduced at breakfast or lunchtime and it's a good idea to serve them for two consecutive days so that your baby becomes familiar with them and if there is a reaction to a food you will know what caused it.

Make the last meal of the day high in carbohydrates: baby rice and mashed banana are ideal choices as they're easily digested and release energy slowly and so should help prevent your baby waking through hunger in the night!

When you reach the end of two weeks, simply start at the beginning again and repeat the meals for another two weeks.

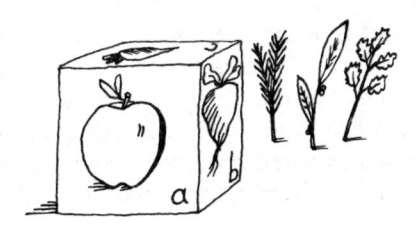

Foods to avoid at five months

- Citrus fruits.
- Cows' milk.
- Eggs.
- Foods containing gluten, found in wheat, including bread and some cereals.
- Honey, as this may contain botulism bacteria.
- Nuts, including peanut butter and sesame seeds.
- Red meat and shellfish.
- Salty and spicy foods.

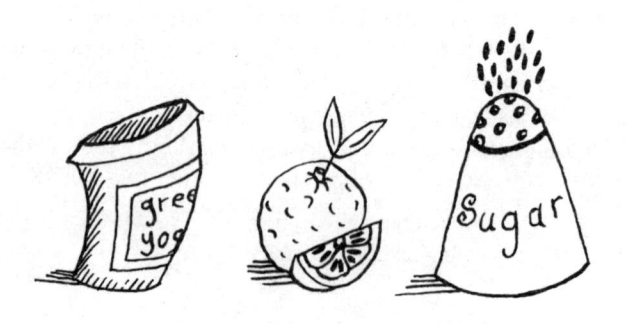

Five to six month meal planner

Day	Breakfast	Lunch	Tea
Week 1			
Monday	Creamed rice with apple (page 47)	Autumn vegetable trio (page 40)	Low-sugar rusk mashed with baby milk
Tuesday	Creamed rice with apple (page 47)	Autumn vegetable trio (page 40)	Mashed banana
Wednesday	Banana and kiwi fruit (page 48)	Cream of pumpkin (page 46)	Baby rice cereal mixed with baby milk
Thursday	Apple and raspberry purée (page 49)	Cream of pumpkin (page 46)	Creamed rice with pear purée (page 31)
Friday	Apple and raspberry purée (page 49)	Red lentils with vegetables (page 39)	Creamed rice with pear purée (page 31)
Saturday	Apricot smoothie (page 50)	Red lentils with vegetables (page 39)	Low-sugar rusk mashed with baby milk
Sunday	Apricot smoothie (page 50)	Chicken casserole (page 41)	Mashed banana

About Five Months

Day Week 2	Breakfast	Lunch	Tea
Monday	Cream of plum and pear (page 51)	Chicken casserole (page 41)	Baby rice cereal mixed with baby milk
Tuesday	Cream of plum and pear (page 51)	Sweet potato and spinach (page 44)	Low-sugar rusk mashed with baby milk
Wednesday	Blushing fruit salad (page 52)	Sweet potato and spinach (page 44)	Mashed banana
Thursday	Blushing fruit salad (page 52)	Cod and courgette savoury (page 42)	Baby rice cereal mixed with baby milk
Friday	Vanilla peach purée (page 53)	Cod and courgette savoury (page 42)	Low-sugar rusk mashed with baby milk
Saturday	Vanilla peach purée (page 53)	Turkey with peas and sweetcorn (page 45)	Mashed banana
Sunday	Banana and kiwi fruit (page 48)	Turkey with peas and sweetcorn (page 45)	Baby rice cereal mixed with baby milk

Red lentils with vegetables

❖ MAKES 4 BABY PORTIONS

15 g/½ oz/1 tbsp red lentils
1 small carrot
100 g/4 oz cauliflower
100 g/4 oz potato
250 ml/8 fl oz/1 cup formula or breast milk

1. Rinse the lentils thoroughly, discarding any black bits. Trim and peel the vegetables and cut into 2.5 cm/1 in dice.

2. Put the lentils and vegetables in a small, heavy-based saucepan with the milk. Bring to the boil, cover and simmer gently for 30 minutes or until the lentils and vegetables are very tender. Check towards the end of the cooking time and top up with a little more milk or boiling water if needed.

3. Purée or sieve (strain) the lentils and vegetables until smooth. Spoon a portion into a bowl and allow to cool, if necessary, before serving.

4. Cool the remaining purée, divide into portions and freeze, or cover and store in the fridge for up to 24 hours.

Tip
The purée will thicken as it cools, so you may need to stir in a little more milk or cooled boiled water before serving.

About Five Months

Autumn vegetable trio

❅ MAKES 4 BABY PORTIONS

1 small carrot
100 g/4 oz potato
100 g/4 oz swede (rutabaga)
150 ml/¼ pint/⅔ cup formula or breast milk

1. Trim and peel the carrot, potato and swede and cut into 2.5 cm/1 in dice. Put the vegetables in a small, heavy-based saucepan and add the milk.

2. Bring the milk to the boil, lower the heat, cover and simmer for 15 minutes or until the vegetables are very soft.

3. Purée or sieve (strain) the vegetables and milk until smooth. Spoon a portion into a bowl and allow to cool, if necessary, before serving.

4. Cool the remaining purée, divide into portions and freeze, or cover and store in the fridge for up to 24 hours.

Tip
Thin the purée with a little extra milk or cooled boiled water if your baby prefers a softer mixture.

Chicken casserole

❦ MAKES 4 BABY PORTIONS

1 small carrot
100 g/4 oz potato
50 g/2 oz chicken breast, skinned and boned
150 ml/¼ pint/⅔ cup vegetable stock (see page 54) or formula or breast milk

1. Trim and peel the carrot and potato and cut into cubes. Cut the chicken into thin strips and put in a small saucepan with the vegetables. Pour in the stock or milk.

2. Bring to the boil, lower the heat, cover and simmer for 15–20 minutes until the chicken and vegetables are cooked.

3. Purée the mixture until smooth. Spoon a portion into a bowl and allow to cool slightly, if necessary, before serving.

4. Cool the remaining purée, divide into portions and freeze, or cover and store in the fridge for up to 24 hours.

Cod and courgette savoury

Cooking fish in foil seals in all the juices and flavour. This is a great way to serve fish and, if cooking for the rest of the family, use cod cutlets and simply add a slice of lemon and a sprig or two of dill, parsley or thyme to their portions.

❈ MAKES 4 BABY PORTIONS

1 small courgette (zucchini)
75 g/3 oz cod fillet, skinned
45 ml/3 tbsp vegetable stock (page 54)
2.5 ml/½ tsp butter or margarine

1 Trim the courgette and cut it into thin slices. Put the fish on a piece of foil, scatter over the courgette, then spoon over the stock. Top with the butter or margarine.

2 Bring the edges of the foil together and fold over to seal and make a parcel. Place on a baking (cookie) sheet.

3 Bake in a preheated oven at 180°C/350°F/gas 4/fan oven 160°C for 20 minutes or until the fish is cooked and the courgette is tender.

4 Flake the fish with a fork, removing any bones, then purée with the courgette and juices until smooth. Spoon a portion into a bowl and allow to cool slightly, if necessary, before serving.

About Five Months

5 Cool the remaining purée, divide into portions and freeze, or cover and store in the fridge for up to 24 hours.

Tip
Add a little more stock or formula or breast milk, if necessary, to make the purée the desired consistency.

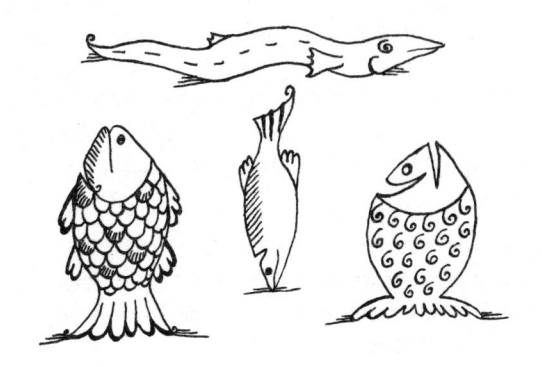

About Five Months

Sweet potato and spinach

❋ MAKES 4 BABY PORTIONS

100 g/4 oz sweet potato
150 ml/¼ pint/⅔ cup formula or breast milk
100 g/4 oz fresh baby spinach leaves

1. Peel and rinse the sweet potato and cut into even-sized pieces. Put in a small saucepan with the milk. Bring to the boil, lower the heat, cover and simmer for 10 minutes.

2. Meanwhile, thoroughly wash the spinach leaves. Remove the excess water in a salad spinner or by patting dry with kitchen paper (paper towels). Remove the stalks.

3. Put the spinach on top of the sweet potato in the pan, cover and cook for a further 8–10 minutes or until the potato and spinach are both very tender.

4. Mash the mixture together until smooth, then press through a sieve (strainer). Spoon a portion into a bowl and allow to cool slightly, if necessary, before serving.

5. Cool the remaining purée, divide into portions and freeze, or cover and store in the fridge for up to 24 hours.

Turkey with peas and sweetcorn

❈ MAKES 4 BABY PORTIONS

100 g/4 oz potato
50 g/2 oz turkey breast, skinned and boned
150 ml/¼ pint/⅔ cup formula or breast milk
25 g/1 oz frozen peas
25 g/1 oz frozen or canned sweetcorn (corn) in water

1. Peel and rinse the potato and cut into even-sized pieces. Cut the turkey into thin strips. Put the potato and turkey in a small saucepan with the milk.

2. Bring to the boil, lower the heat, cover and simmer for 10 minutes. Add the peas and sweetcorn and cook for a further 5–10 minutes until the turkey and vegetables are cooked.

3. Purée the mixture until smooth. Spoon a portion into a bowl and allow to cool slightly, if necessary, before serving.

4. Cool the remaining purée, divide into portions and freeze, or cover and store in the fridge for up to 24 hours.

About Five Months

Cream of pumpkin

❋ MAKES 4 BABY PORTIONS

100 g/4 oz pumpkin
10 ml/2 tsp baby rice
120 ml/4 fl oz/½ cup warm formula or breast milk

1. Thickly peel the pumpkin and remove the seeds. Cut the flesh into dice. Put in a steamer or in a sieve (strainer) over a pan of boiling water and cover with a lid.

2. Steam the pumpkin for about 8 minutes or until very tender. Purée in a blender or press through a fine sieve.

3. Mix the baby rice with the milk until smooth. Stir in the pumpkin purée. Spoon a portion into a bowl and allow to cool, if necessary.

4. Cool the remainder, divide into portions and freeze, or cover and store in the fridge for up to 24 hours.

Creamed rice with apple

MAKES 2 BABY PORTIONS

½ sweet eating (dessert) apple
15 ml/1 tbsp flaked rice
100 ml/3½ fl oz/scant ½ cup formula or breast milk

1 Quarter, core and peel the apple. Slice thinly and put in a small saucepan with the rice and milk.

2 Bring to the boil, cover, then simmer very gently for 12–15 minutes, stirring occasionally, until the apple and rice are cooked.

3 Purée the mixture until smooth. Spoon half into a bowl and allow to cool slightly, if necessary, before serving.

4 Cool the remaining purée, cover and store in the fridge for up to 24 hours.

Tip
For Creamed Rice with Pear, replace the apple with pear.

About Five Months

Banana and kiwi fruit

MAKES 1 BABY PORTION

¼ ripe banana
¼ ripe kiwi fruit

1. Remove the peel from the banana and kiwi fruit. Mash the banana with a fork until smooth, then push through a fine sieve (strainer).
2. Mash the kiwi fruit and push through the sieve to remove the black pips.
3. Mix the two purées together and serve straight away.

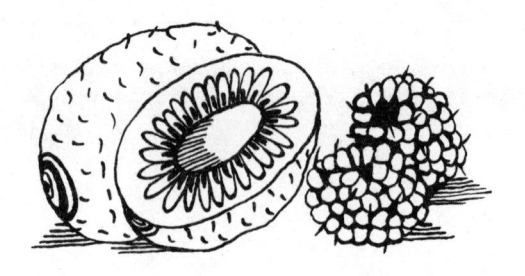

Apple and raspberry purée

❊ MAKES 4 BABY PORTIONS

1 eating (dessert) apple
15 ml/1 tbsp apple juice or water
25 g/1 oz fresh or frozen raspberries

1. Quarter, core, peel and thinly slice the apple. Put in a small saucepan with the apple juice or water.

2. Cover and cook over a very low heat for 5 minutes. Add the raspberries and cook for a further 3–4 minutes, stirring occasionally, until the fruit is very soft.

3. Press the mixture through a sieve (strainer) or purée in a blender. If you have used a blender, rub the purée through a sieve to remove the berry pips. Spoon a portion into a bowl and allow to cool slightly, if necessary, before serving.

4. Cool the remaining purée, divide into portions and freeze, or cover and store in the fridge for up to 24 hours.

Apricot smoothie

Mixing a more strongly flavoured fruit, such as apricot, with baby rice makes it more palatable when introducing a new taste.

MAKES 2 BABY PORTIONS

1 ripe apricot
5 ml/1 tsp water
10 ml/2 tsp baby rice
20 ml/4 tsp formula or breast milk

1. Halve the apricot, discard the stone (pit), then chop the flesh roughly. Put in a small saucepan with the water. Cover and simmer gently for 8 minutes or until the fruit is soft.

2. Sieve (strain) the fruit to remove the skin. Blend the baby rice with the milk, then stir in the fruit purée. Spoon a portion into a bowl and allow to cool slightly, if necessary, before serving.

3. Cool the remaining mixture, cover and store in the fridge for up to 24 hours.

Tip
If fresh apricots aren't in season, use 2 canned apricot halves in natural juice rather than in syrup. They will need cooking for only 2–3 minutes at step 1.

Cream of plum and pear

❉ MAKES 4 BABY PORTIONS

1 ripe plum
½ ripe pear
10 ml/2 tsp apple juice or water
½ low-sugar rusk
30 ml/2 tbsp formula or breast milk

1. Peel the plum (see method for Vanilla Peach Purée on page 53 if the skin is difficult to remove). Cut in half and remove the stone (pit). Quarter, core and peel the pear. Roughly chop the fruit and put in a small saucepan with the apple juice or water.

2. Cover and simmer gently for 10 minutes until very soft, stirring occasionally. Sieve (strain) or purée the fruit until smooth.

3. Meanwhile, crumble the rusk into a bowl and sprinkle over the milk. Leave to soften for a few minutes, then mix until smooth. Stir in the fruit purée.

4. Spoon a portion into a bowl and allow to cool slightly, if necessary, before serving.

5. Cool the remaining mixture, divide into portions and freeze, or cover and store in the fridge for up to 24 hours.

Blushing fruit salad

❋ MAKES 4 BABY PORTIONS

½ ripe pear
10 ml/2 tsp apple juice or water
¼ charentais melon
25 g/1 oz fresh or frozen raspberries

1. Quarter, core and peel the pear. Cut into thin slices. Put in a small saucepan with the apple juice or water and simmer gently for 5 minutes.

2. Meanwhile, scoop the seeds out of the melon, cut off the skin and dice the flesh. Add to the pan with the raspberries and cook for a further 3–4 minutes until the fruit is soft.

3. Press the mixture though a sieve (strainer) or purée in a blender and then sieve (strain) to remove the berry pips.

4. Spoon a portion into a bowl and allow to cool slightly, if necessary, before serving.

5. Cool the remaining purée, divide into portions and freeze, or cover and store in the fridge for up to 24 hours.

Vanilla peach purée

❋ MAKES 4 BABY PORTIONS

1 ripe peach or nectarine
2.5 cm/1 in piece of vanilla pod
15 ml/1 tbsp peach or apple juice or water

1. Peel the peach or nectarine. If this is difficult, put in a bowl and cover with boiling water. Remove after 1 minute and rinse under cold water. The skin should come away easily.

2. Halve the fruit, remove the stone (pit), then chop the flesh and put in a small saucepan with the vanilla pod and juice or water. Cover the pan and cook over a low heat for 10 minutes until the fruit is tender. Remove the vanilla pod.

3. Sieve (strain) or purée the fruit until smooth. Spoon a portion into a bowl and allow to cool slightly, if necessary, before serving.

4. Cool the remaining purée, divide into portions and freeze, or cover and store in the fridge for up to 24 hours.

Tip
Don't throw away the piece of vanilla pod after using. Rinse under cold running water, leave to dry, then store in an airtight container. It can be re-used several times. If you prefer, the peach purée can be made without the vanilla.

About Five Months

Home-made vegetable stock

Throughout this and subsequent chapters, you'll find recipes that call for vegetable stock. Don't use commercial stock (bouillon) cubes, granules or powder until your baby is at least nine months old and then only in small amounts, as they contain large quantities of salt. Adding salt puts a strain on the baby's kidneys and encourages a taste for salt, rather than the natural flavour of food, to develop. If you haven't got time to make stock, water may be used in the recipes instead.

❊ MAKES 600 ML/1 PINT/2½ CUPS

1 onion, peeled
2 celery sticks
2 carrots, peeled
900 ml/1½ pints/3¾ cups water
2 bay leaves
A few fresh parsley or thyme sprigs

1 Roughly chop the onion, celery and carrots. Put in a saucepan with the water and herbs.

2 Slowly bring to the boil and skim the surface. Part-cover the pan with a lid and simmer for 40 minutes. Leave to cool.

3. Strain the stock through a fine sieve (strainer), discarding the vegetables and herbs. Cover and store in the fridge for up to 3 days or freeze for up to 3 months.

Tip
You'll need different amounts of stock for the recipes, so freeze some 15 ml/1 tbsp portions in sterilised ice cube trays and some 150 ml/¼ pint/⅔ cup portions in suitable containers.

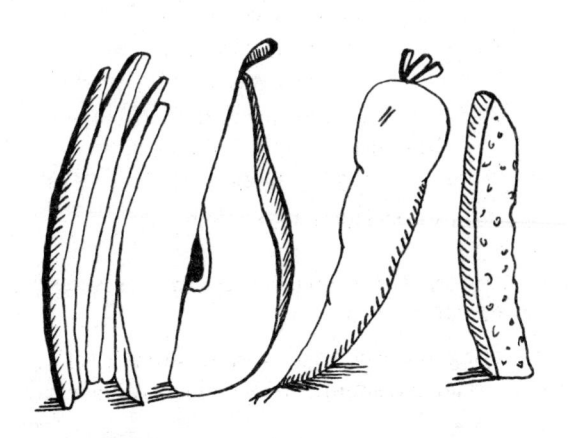

Six to Nine Months

Your baby can now move on to slightly more textured puréed or mashed food. Try keeping it fairly soft at first, with just a few small lumps, but allow your baby to guide you – some are very resistant to even the tiniest piece! By now she'll have preferences for certain foods and perhaps a few dislikes as well. You can still serve the meals in the previous chapter – choose those she's familiar with and enjoys, but make them very slightly coarser to get her used to a lumpier texture. There are plenty of new recipes to try in this chapter, but no day-by-day menu planner; it will benefit your baby (and you'll find it a lot easier) if she can start to join in with suitable family meals at this age.

You can use full-fat cows' milk or formula milk in cooking from this age, but stick to formula or breast milk for drinking.

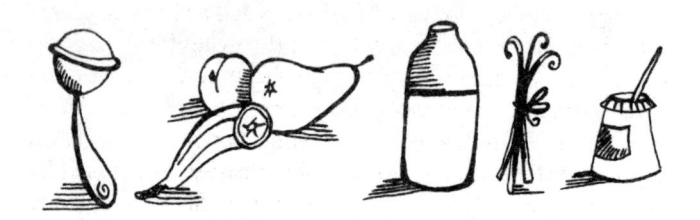

Self-feeding

At around six or seven months, your baby will probably take the first steps towards self-feeding. This is a vital step in her development, so don't discourage her and be prepared to cope with lots of mess to begin with. Gradually she'll become adept at feeding herself and the sooner you start, the quicker you'll reach this stage. She may start grabbing the spoon, so try giving her a second (identical) spoon to hold while you feed her. It will be a couple months, or even longer before she's really able to feed herself, but once she can get the spoon from the bowl and into her mouth, you can help by giving foods that will stick to the spoon rather than slipping straight off – porridge works particularly well. Try introducing a few simple finger foods, such as sticks of lightly cooked vegetables (not raw at this stage) or breadsticks to suck; they encourage independence and will hopefully give you a chance to enjoy your own meal. By nine months your baby should be able to cope with a range of finger foods and you'll find a list of these in the next chapter.

When your baby begins to feed herself, eating will take a lot longer, so try to allow for this. Meal times will be seen as a game and this may include playing with and throwing food. She will probably use her fingers, rather than the spoon, at times and enjoy smearing the food around the tray; try to ignore this as long as she is eating as well as playing, but if she's finished eating, remove the food at once. Make it easier on yourself by surrounding the highchair with newspaper. She's also ready

Six to Nine Months

now to use a trainer cup by herself. Choose a plastic one that's less likely to break when dropped or thrown and make sure that the lid is secure.

What to do if your child chokes

Never leave your child alone while eating; it's essential that you are there to react quickly if she gags or chokes. If she splutters and gags while eating but can still breathe, reassure her by patting her firmly on the back and talking to her calmly.

If she can't breathe or cough, the windpipe is blocked and you need to take immediate action. Tip her up so that her head is lower than her chest, supporting her head with your forearm and slap firmly between the shoulder blades. If the food is coughed up into her mouth, remove it while her head is still down to prevent re-inhalation. If this does not work, sit the baby up and look down her throat. If you can see the offending object, try to hook it out with your finger (the baby will probably retch, but don't worry as this may help push the trapped object forward). If you're still unsuccessful, don't hesitate to ring for the emergency services, still holding her head downwards.

Foods to avoid from six to nine months

- Egg white.
- Salty, very spicy and sugary foods, including honey.
- Shellfish.
- Nuts, including peanut butter and sesame seeds.

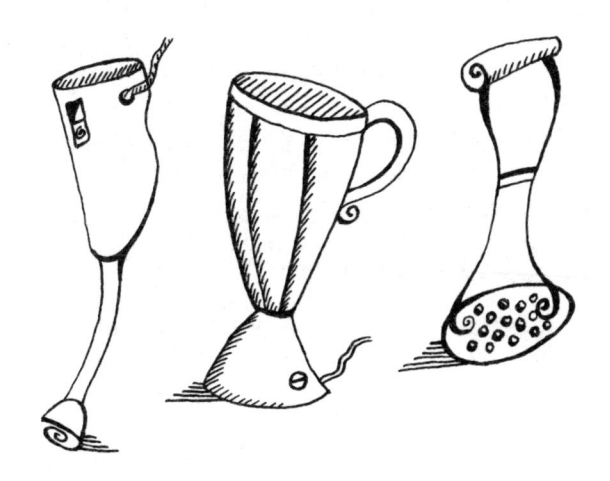

Mixed vegetable risotto

❋ MAKES 6 BABY PORTIONS

50 g/2 oz/¼ cup long-grain rice
¼ small red (bell) pepper
25 g/1 oz frozen mixed vegetables
300 ml/½ pint/1¼ cups milk

1. Rinse the rice under cold running water and put in a small saucepan. Trim the pepper and dice the flesh. Add the pepper and mixed vegetables to the rice and pour in the milk.

2. Bring to the boil, part-cover the pan with a lid and simmer for about 12 minutes or until the rice and vegetables are soft.

3. Purée the mixture until fairly smooth. Spoon a portion into a bowl and allow to cool slightly, if necessary, before serving.

4. Cool the remaining purée, divide into portions and freeze, or cover and store in the fridge for up to 24 hours.

Creamed cod and corn chowder

❀ MAKES 6 BABY PORTIONS

100 g/4 oz skinless cod fillet
300 ml/½ pint/1¼ cups milk
75 g/3 oz sweet potato
50 g/2 oz canned or frozen sweetcorn (corn) in water
1 sprig of fresh parsley, stalk removed (optional)

1. Put the fish in a small pan with the milk. Slowly bring to a simmer and poach for 7–8 minutes or until the fish is cooked. Remove the fish from the pan, using a slotted spoon, flake into pieces, taking care to remove any bones, and set aside. Reserve the milk.

2. Meanwhile, peel the sweet potato and cut into 2.5 cm/1 in dice. Add to the milk. Bring to the boil and simmer for 10 minutes. Add the sweetcorn and parsley and cook for a further 5 minutes or until the sweet potato is very tender.

3. Purée the vegetable and milk mixture with the fish until fairly smooth. Spoon a portion into a bowl and allow to cool slightly, if necessary, before serving.

4. Cool the remaining purée, divide into portions and freeze, or cover and store in the fridge for up to 24 hours.

Chicken with garden vegetables

❊ MAKES 6 BABY PORTIONS

1 small carrot
100 g/4 oz potato
4 green (French) beans
100 g/4 oz chicken breast, skinned and boned
150 ml/¼ pint/⅔ cup milk

1 Trim and peel the carrot and potato and cut into small cubes. Trim the beans and cut each into three or four pieces. Slice the chicken into thin strips. Put in a small saucepan with the vegetables and add the milk.

2 Part-cover the pan with a lid and simmer for 15 minutes or until the chicken and vegetables are cooked.

3 Purée the mixture until fairly smooth. Spoon a portion into a bowl and allow to cool, if necessary, before serving.

4 Cool the remaining purée, divide into portions and freeze, or cover and store in the fridge for up to 24 hours.

One-pot chicken and rice

❋ MAKES 6 BABY PORTIONS

50 g/2 oz /¼ cup long-grain rice
300 ml/½ pint/1¼ cups milk
100 g/4 oz chicken breast, skinned and boned
1 small carrot
100 g/4 oz broccoli

1. Rinse the rice under cold running water and put in a small saucepan with the milk.

2. Cut the chicken into thin strips. Trim, peel and slice the carrot. Divide the broccoli into small florets. Add to the pan and bring to the boil.

3. Stir, then part-cover the pan with a lid and simmer for 12–15 minutes or until the rice and vegetables are soft.

4. Purée the mixture until fairly smooth. Spoon a portion into a bowl and allow to cool slightly, if necessary, before serving.

5. Cool the remaining purée, divide into portions and freeze, or cover and store in the fridge for up to 24 hours.

Broccoli and cauliflower cheese

Serve this vegetable dish as part the family meal. Remember to remove a couple of portions for baby before seasoning.

❋ MAKES 2 ADULT PLUS 2 BABY PORTIONS

½ medium cauliflower, cut into florets
225 g/8 oz broccoli, cut into florets
40 g/1½ oz/scant ¼ cup butter or margarine
45 ml/3 tbsp plain (all-purpose) flour
1 bay leaf
300 ml/½ pint/1¼ cups milk
75 g/3 oz/¾ cup freshly grated mild or medium Cheddar cheese

1. Bring a pan of water to the boil and add the cauliflower and broccoli. Cover and simmer for 10 minutes or until tender. Alternatively, put in a steamer over boiling water and cook for 12 minutes.

2. Meanwhile, put the butter or margarine, flour, bay leaf and milk in a small saucepan. Slowly bring to the boil, stirring all the time, until the sauce thickens. Turn down the heat and simmer for 3 minutes. Discard the bay leaf.

3 Remove the sauce from the heat and stir in the cheese until melted.

4 Remove three florets each of the cauliflower and broccoli and about 60 ml/4 tbsp of the sauce. (The remainder will serve two adults.) Mash together with a fork or purée until fairly smooth, adding a little extra milk if needed.

5 Spoon half the purée into a bowl and allow to cool slightly, if necessary, before serving.

6 Cool the remaining portion and freeze, or cover and store in the fridge for up to 24 hours.

Tip
If you prefer, make half the quantity of this recipe and divide into six portions for baby meals.

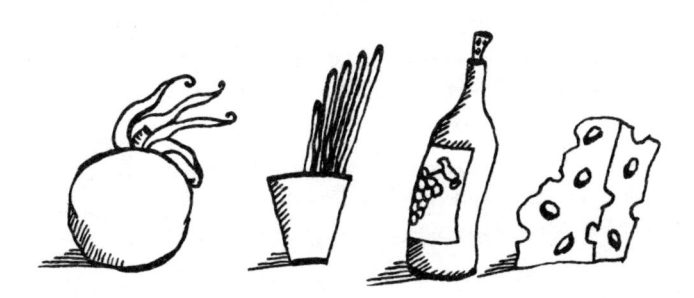

Beef and carrot braise

❋ MAKES 6 BABY PORTIONS

100 g/4 oz lean stewing beef
15 ml/1 tbsp sunflower oil
4 spring onions (scallions)
1 medium carrot
175 g/6 oz potatoes
1.5 ml/¼ tsp yeast extract, such as Marmite
A pinch of dried mixed herbs
300 ml/½ pint/1¼ cups hot vegetable stock (see page 54)
or water

1. Trim any fat or gristle from the beef and cut the meat into small cubes. Heat the oil in a small flameproof casserole dish (Dutch oven), add the beef and fry (sauté) until lightly browned. Remove from the heat.

2. Trim the spring onions and cut them into 2.5 cm/1 in lengths. Trim and peel the carrot and potatoes. Cut the vegetables into large cubes and add to the casserole dish.

3. Stir the yeast extract and herbs into the hot vegetable stock or water and pour over the meat and vegetables.

Six to Nine Months

4. Cover the casserole and simmer very gently for about 1 hour or until the meat is tender. Alternatively, cook in a preheated oven at 180°C/350°F/gas 4/fan oven 160°C for 1½ hours.

5. Purée the mixture until fairly smooth. Spoon a portion into a bowl and allow to cool slightly, if necessary, before serving.

6. Cool the remaining purée, divide into portions and freeze, or cover and store in the fridge for up to 24 hours.

Tip
Yeast extract is very salty so don't be tempted to add more than the recipe states.

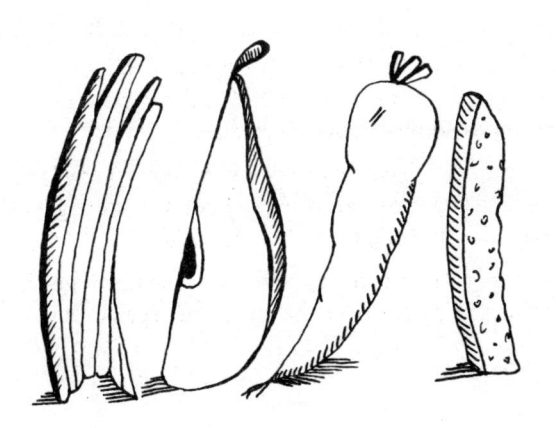

Savoury pork and apple casserole

❀ MAKES 6 BABY PORTIONS

100 g/4 oz lean pork, such as tenderloin
100 g/4 oz potato
100 g/4 oz parsnip
1 small eating (dessert) apple
A pinch of dried mixed herbs
300 ml/½ pint/1¼ cups vegetable stock (see page 54)
or water

1. Trim any fat or gristle from the pork and slice thinly. Peel the potato and parsnip and cut into chunks. Peel, quarter and core the apple and roughly chop.

2. Put the meat, vegetables, apple, herbs and stock or water in a small pan. Bring to the boil, cover and simmer gently for about 45 minutes or until the meat is tender. Alternatively, cook in a preheated oven at 180°C/350°F/gas 4/fan oven 160°C for 1¼ hours.

3. Purée the mixture until fairly smooth. Spoon a portion into a bowl and allow to cool slightly, if necessary, before serving.

4 Cool the remaining purée, divide into portions and freeze, or cover and store in the fridge for up to 24 hours.

Tip
The parsnip can be replaced with another root vegetable such as swede (rutabaga) or carrot.

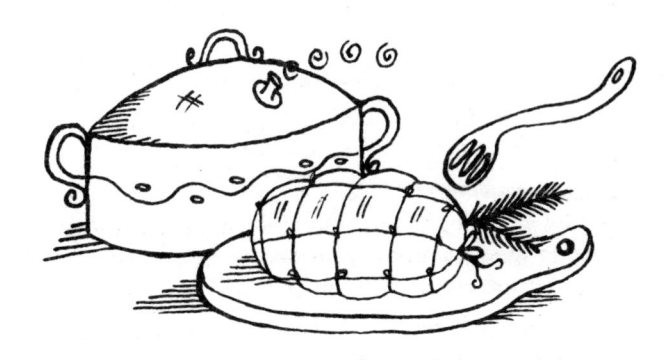

Poached fish with pea and potato purée

❁ MAKES 4 BABY PORTIONS

100 g/4 oz plaice fillet, skinned
1 bay leaf
150 ml/¼ pint/⅔ cup milk
100 g/4 oz potato
25 g/1 oz frozen peas
5 ml/1 tsp snipped fresh chives or chopped fresh parsley (optional)

1. Put the fish in a small saucepan with the bay leaf. Pour over the milk. Slowly bring to the boil, part-cover the pan with a lid and simmer for 10–12 minutes or until the fish is cooked.

2. Remove the fish from the milk using a slotted spoon, then flake the flesh and roughly mash with a fork, removing any bones. Discard the bay leaf and reserve the milk.

3. Meanwhile, peel the potato and cut into chunks. Cook in boiling water for 10 minutes. Add the peas and cook for a further 5 minutes or until the potato is tender. Drain well.

Six to Nine Months

4. Mash the potato and peas with enough of the reserved milk to make a smooth mixture. Stir in the fish and herbs, if using.

5. Spoon a portion into a bowl and allow to cool slightly, if necessary, before serving.

6. Cool the remaining purée, divide into portions and freeze, or cover and store in the fridge for up to 24 hours.

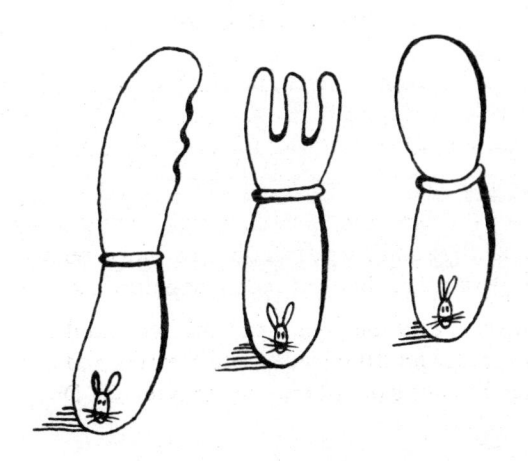

Creamed potato and celeriac with cheese

You can also turn this vegetable purée into a delicious dish for two or three adults to accompany chicken or game by seasoning with salt, black pepper and plenty of freshly grated nutmeg after removing a portion for baby.

❋ MAKES 4 BABY PORTIONS

175 g/6 oz potatoes
175 g/6 oz celeriac (celery root)
25 g/1 oz/2 tbsp butter or margarine
75 ml/5 tbsp milk
15 g/½ oz/1 tbsp finely grated mild Cheddar cheese

1. Peel the potatoes and celeriac and cut into large chunks. Cook in boiling water for 15 minutes or until very tender. Drain well.

2. Mash the vegetables together with the butter or margarine and milk until smooth, adding a little more milk if needed.

3. Spoon a portion into a bowl. Allow it to cool slightly, if necessary, stir in the cheese, then serve.

4. Cool the remaining purée, divide into portions and freeze, or cover and store in the fridge for up to 24 hours.

Tip
Don't add the cheese before freezing the vegetable purée, as it tends to go stringy when reheated.

Cream of carrot and courgette

MAKES 2 BABY PORTIONS

1 medium carrot
½ small courgette (zucchini)
75 ml/5 tbsp warm milk
15 ml/1 tbsp baby rice

1. Trim, peel and slice the carrot. Wash, trim and slice the courgette. Put in a steamer or a sieve (strainer) placed over a pan of boiling water, and cook for about 15 minutes or until very soft.

2. Purée the vegetables with 60 ml/4 tbsp of the milk until fairly smooth.

3. Blend the rice and remaining milk together, then stir in the puréed vegetables.

4. Spoon half the purée into a bowl and allow to cool slightly, if necessary, before serving.

5. Cool the remaining purée, cover and store in the fridge for up to 24 hours.

Creamy carrot and coriander with lentils

❀ MAKES 4 BABY PORTIONS

3 medium carrots
50 g/2 oz/⅓ cup red lentils
200 ml /7 fl oz/scant 1 cup milk
2.5 ml/½ tsp chopped fresh coriander (cilantro)

1. Trim, peel and slice the carrots and put in a small saucepan. Rinse and pick over the lentils. Add to the pan with the milk.

2. Bring to the boil, turn down the heat, cover and simmer for about 30 minutes or until the lentils are very soft. Stir in the coriander.

3. Sieve (strain) or purée the mixture until fairly smooth. Spoon a portion into a bowl and allow to cool slightly, if necessary, before serving.

4. Cool the remaining purée, divide into portions and freeze, or cover and store in the fridge for up to 24 hours.

Tip
You can use fresh parsley instead of the coriander, or leave it out altogether if preferred.

Quick fish kedgeree

❇ MAKES 6 BABY PORTIONS

50 g/2 oz/¼ cup long-grain rice
100 g/4 oz frozen skinless cod fillet
300 ml/½ pint/1¼ cups milk
1 hard-boiled (hard-cooked) egg yolk
10 ml/2 tsp chopped fresh parsley

1. Rinse the rice under cold running water. Put it in a small saucepan with the cod and milk. Bring to the boil, part-cover the pan with a lid and simmer for 15 minutes or until the rice and fish are cooked.

2. Remove the fish from the pan and flake with a fork, removing any bones. Stir the fish into the rice with the egg yolk and parsley. Mash or purée the mixture until fairly smooth.

3. Spoon a portion into a bowl and allow to cool slightly, if necessary, before serving.

4. Cool the remaining mixture, divide into portions and freeze, or cover and store in the fridge for up to 24 hours.

Leek and potato purée

To turn this into a tasty soup for 3–4 adults, double the quantity, season and thin down with extra stock or milk and serve topped with crème fraîche and a sprinkling of snipped fresh chives.

❋ MAKES 6 BABY PORTIONS

175 g/6 oz small or baby leeks
25 g/1 oz/2 tbsp butter or margarine
100 g/4 oz floury potatoes
1 bay leaf
120 ml/4 fl oz/½ cup vegetable stock (see page 54)
120 ml/4 fl oz/½ cup milk
To serve:
Plain fromage frais

1. Trim and thoroughly wash the leeks. Cut into thin slices.
2. Melt the butter or margarine in a saucepan. Add the leeks and cook over a gentle heat for 10 minutes until soft.
3. Meanwhile, peel the potatoes and cut into chunks. Add the potato chunks to the leeks with the bay leaf, stock and milk. Bring to the boil, lower the heat, cover and simmer for 20 minutes until the potatoes are tender.

Six to Nine Months

4 Discard the bay leaf. Purée the vegetable mixture until fairly smooth. Spoon a portion into a bowl and allow to cool slightly if necessary. Stir in 30 ml/2 tbsp of fromage frais before serving.

5 Cool the remaining purée, divide into portions and freeze, or cover and store in the fridge for up to 24 hours.

Tips
Freeze without the fromage frais. Use all milk instead of a mixture of stock and milk, if preferred.

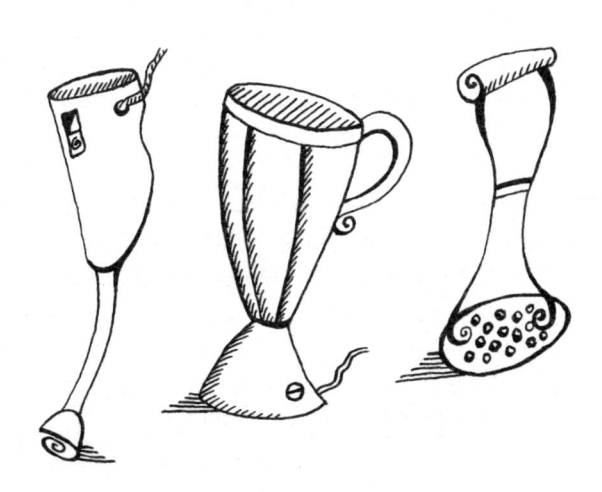

Potato and watercress purée with fromage frais

MAKES 2 BABY PORTIONS

100 g/4 oz potato
2 or 3 sprigs of watercress
15 g/½ oz/1 tbsp butter or margarine
60 ml/4 tbsp plain fromage frais

1. Peel the potato and cut into chunks. Cook in boiling water for 15 minutes or until tender. Drain well.

2. Meanwhile, remove the tough stems from the watercress and finely chop the leaves. Melt the butter or margarine in a small pan and gently cook the watercress for about 2 minutes until wilted and tender.

3. Mash the potato with the watercress, butter or margarine and fromage frais until smooth. Spoon half into a bowl and allow to cool slightly, if necessary, before serving.

4. Cool the remaining mixture, cover and store in the fridge for up to 24 hours.

Vegetable medley

❊ MAKES 6 BABY PORTIONS

100 g/4 oz swede (rutabaga)
100 g/4 oz potato
100 g/4 oz broccoli
50 g/2 oz green cabbage
250 ml/8 fl oz/1 cup milk

1. Peel and dice the swede and potato. Cut the broccoli into florets and finely shred the cabbage. Put the vegetables in a small saucepan with the milk.

2. Bring to the boil, lower the heat and cook, part-covered, for 12–15 minutes until all the vegetables are very tender.

3. Sieve (strain) or purée the mixture until fairly smooth. Spoon a portion into a bowl and allow to cool slightly, if necessary, before serving.

4. Cool the remaining purée, divide into portions and freeze, or cover and store in the fridge for up to 24 hours.

Mediterranean vegetables with pasta

❀ MAKES 6 BABY PORTIONS

2 ripe tomatoes
1 small courgette (zucchini)
100 g/4 oz red (bell) pepper
5 ml/1 tsp tomato purée (paste)
175 ml/6 fl oz/¾ cup vegetable stock (see page 54) or water
A small pinch of dried basil or dried mixed herbs
25 g/1 oz mini pasta shapes

1. Plunge the tomatoes into boiling water for 1 minute, then remove, rinse under cold water and peel off the skins, then quarter and remove the seeds.

2. Rinse, trim and slice the courgette. Cut away the core and seeds from the pepper, then chop the flesh. Put the vegetables in a saucepan with the tomato purée, stock or water and herbs. Cover and simmer for 10 minutes.

3. Add the pasta and cook for a further 5 minutes or until the vegetables and pasta are very soft.

4. Purée or mash the mixture with a fork until fairly smooth. Spoon a portion into a bowl and allow to cool slightly, if necessary, before serving.

5. Cool the remaining purée, divide into portions and freeze, or cover and store in the fridge for up to 24 hours.

Tip
You can buy tiny pasta shapes, usually labelled 'mini' or 'soup' pasta, such as farfalline, which are ideal baby food as they don't need to be chewed.

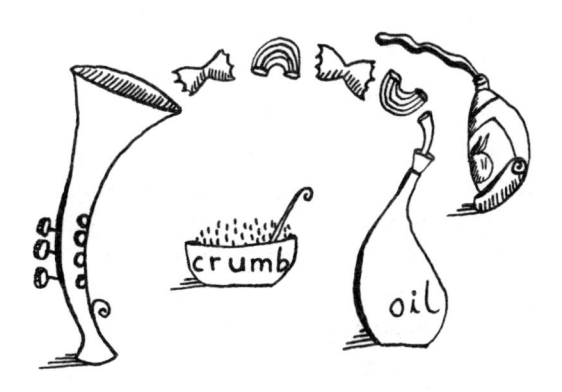

Chocolate rice pudding

MAKES 2 BABY PORTIONS

30 ml /2 tbsp flaked rice
150 ml/¼ pint/⅔ cup milk
25 g/1 oz milk chocolate

1. Place the flaked rice and milk in a small saucepan. Bring to the boil and simmer over a gentle heat for 10 minutes, stirring occasionally, until the rice is cooked. Remove from the heat.

2. Roughly chop the chocolate and add to the hot rice. Stir until melted. Spoon half into a bowl and allow to cool slightly, if necessary, before serving.

3. Cool the remaining portion, cover and store in the fridge for up to 24 hours.

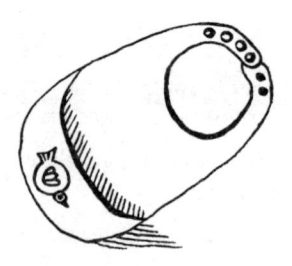

Baked sweet potato and apple

❋ MAKES 6 BABY PORTIONS

1 medium sweet potato
1 eating (dessert) apple
15 g/½ oz/1 tbsp butter or margarine
45 ml/3 tbsp milk
A small pinch of ground cinnamon

1. Gently scrub the sweet potato. Cut a thin slice from the base of the apple so that it stands upright.

2. Prick the sweet potato and apple several times with a fork or skewer, place in an ovenproof dish and loosely cover with foil. Bake in a preheated oven at 180°C/350°F/gas 4/ fan oven 160°C for 40–50 minutes or until tender. Leave until cool enough to handle.

3. Halve the sweet potato and scoop out the flesh. Mash with the butter or margarine, milk and cinnamon until smooth.

4. Halve the apple and remove the core and pips. Scoop out the flesh and add to the potato mixture . Mash until mixed.

5. Spoon a portion into a bowl and allow to cool slightly, if necessary, before serving.

6. Cool the remaining purée and freeze, or cover and store in the fridge for up to 24 hours.

Pear and prune custard

❋ MAKES 6 BABY PORTIONS

2 prunes
75 ml /5 tbsp apple juice or water
1 ripe pear
15 ml/1 tbsp custard powder
5 ml/1 tsp caster (superfine) sugar
150 ml/¼ pint/⅔ cup milk

1. Halve the prunes and remove the stones (pits). Put them in a small bowl with the apple juice or water and leave to soak for at least 4 hours or overnight.

2. Peel, quarter, core and slice the pear. Put it in a small saucepan with the prunes and soaking liquid. Cover and simmer for 10 minutes until soft, stirring occasionally. Rub the fruit through a sieve (strainer) to remove the tough prune skins.

3. Meanwhile, blend the custard powder with the sugar and 30 ml/2 tbsp of the milk. Heat the remaining milk in a pan until boiling, then pour over the custard and milk paste, stirring. Return to the pan and simmer for 1 minute, stirring continuously, until thickened and smooth.

Six to Nine Months

4 Stir the fruit purée into the custard. Spoon a portion into a bowl and allow to cool slightly, if necessary, before serving.

5 Cool the remaining custard, divide into portions and freeze, or cover and store in the fridge for up to 24 hours.

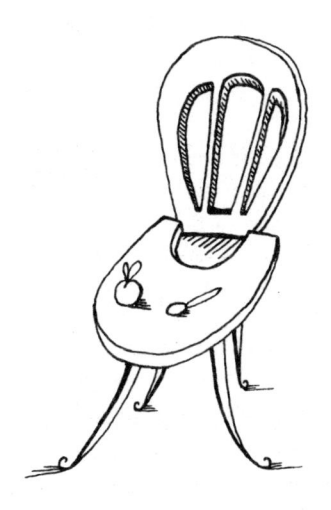

Apple and raspberry ripple yoghurt

❋ MAKES 4 BABY PORTIONS

1 eating (dessert) apple
15 ml/1 tbsp apple juice or water
25 g/1 oz fresh or frozen raspberries
To serve:
Plain Greek yoghurt

1. Peel, quarter and core the apple, then slice it thinly. Put in a small saucepan with the apple juice or water, cover and simmer gently for 5 minutes. Add the raspberries and cook for a further 5 minutes or until very soft.

2. Mash the fruit with a fork, then press though a fine sieve (strainer) to remove the berry pips. Leave the purée to cool.

3. Spoon a quarter of the purée into a bowl. Divide the rest into portions and freeze, or cover and store in the fridge for up to 24 hours.

4. Add 10 ml/2 tsp of yoghurt to the portion of fruit purée and stir to achieve a rippled effect. Serve straight away.

Tip
Freeze without the yoghurt.

Blushing pear dessert

Strawberries or raspberries work equally well in this recipe.

❀ MAKES 4 BABY PORTIONS

1 ripe pear
25 g/1 oz fresh or frozen blackberries
15 ml/1 tbsp orange juice
To serve:
Fromage frais

1. Quarter, core and peel the pear. Slice thinly and put in a small saucepan with the blackberries and orange juice. Cover and simmer for 10 minutes until very soft.

2. Press the mixture through a sieve (strainer) to remove the berry pips.

3. Spoon a quarter of the purée into a bowl. When cool, stir in 10 ml/2 tsp of fromage frais and serve straight away.

4. Cool the remaining fruit purée, divide into portions and freeze, or cover and store in the fridge for up to 24 hours.

Tip
Freeze without the fromage frais.

Banana cream

MAKES 1 PORTION

½ ripe banana
40 g/1½ oz silken tofu
30 ml/2 tbsp orange juice

1. Peel and roughly chop the banana. Put in a food processor with the tofu and orange juice and blend to a smooth purée.

2. Spoon into a bowl and serve straight away, or cover and chill in the fridge for up to 4 hours.

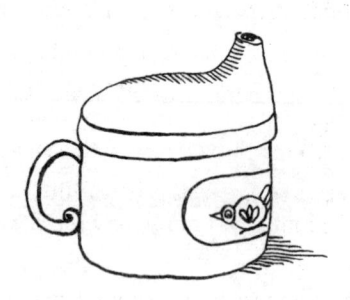

Baked egg custard

Babies shouldn't be given egg whites until they're at least nine months old, so this custard is made with just the yolk.

MAKES 2 BABY PORTIONS

1 egg yolk
2.5 ml/½ tsp cornflour (cornstarch)
5 ml/1 tsp caster (superfine) sugar
A few drops of vanilla essence (extract)
175 ml/6 fl oz/¾ cup milk

1 Blend the egg yolk with the cornflour, sugar and vanilla essence in a bowl. Heat the milk to boiling point, then pour over the egg mixture, whisking all the time.

2 Pour the mixture into two small greased ramekins (custard cups). Place them in a roasting tin (pan) or ovenproof dish and pour enough water into the tin to come half way up the sides of the ramekins. Cover each with a small piece of foil.

3 Bake in a preheated oven at 150°C/300°F/gas 2/fan oven 135°C for 35 minutes or until lightly set. Serve one portion warm or cold.

4 Allow the remaining portion to cool. Cover and chill in the fridge for up to 24 hours to serve cold. (You can take the chill off by leaving it at room temperature for 30 minutes.) Do not reheat.

Orchard fruit fool

❄ MAKES 6 BABY PORTIONS

1 eating (dessert) apple
2 ripe plums
15 ml/1 tbsp apple or orange juice
15 ml/1 tbsp custard powder
10 ml/2 tsp soft light brown sugar
150 ml/¼ pint/⅔ cup milk

1. Quarter, core and peel the apple. Halve the plums, remove the stones (pits) and peel off the skins. Roughly chop the fruit and put in a small saucepan with the apple or orange juice.

2. Cover and simmer for 10 minutes or until the fruit is very tender. Mash with a fork until fairly smooth.

3. Meanwhile, blend the custard powder with the sugar and 30 ml/2 tbsp of the milk until smooth. Heat the remaining milk to boiling point and pour over the custard and milk paste, stirring.

4. Return the custard to the pan and simmer, stirring for 1 minute, until thickened and smooth. Stir in the fruit purée.

5 Spoon a portion into a bowl and allow to cool slightly, if necessary, before serving.

6 Cool the remaining mixture, divide into portions and freeze, or cover and store in the fridge for up to 24 hours.

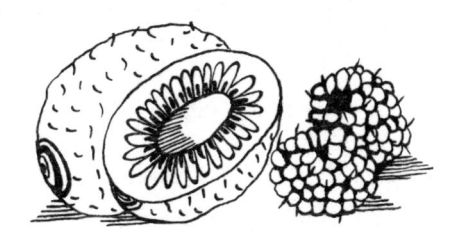

Teething rusks

Most commercial baby rusks contain a large amount of sugar, which can decay teeth as they start to come through. Try these savoury toasts as a simple and inexpensive alternative.

MAKES 8

1.5 ml/¼ tsp yeast extract, such as Marmite
15 ml/1 tbsp boiling water
2 slices of white bread

1. Mix together the yeast extract and water until blended. Very lightly brush the mixture over one side of each slice of bread.

2. Trim the crusts off the bread and cut each slice into four fingers. Bake in a preheated oven at 160°C/325°F/gas mark 3/fan oven 145°C for 25 minutes or until crisp and dry.

3. Leave to cool on a wire rack. Transfer to an airtight container and store for up to 5 days.

Nine to Twelve Months

Your baby will now be eating slightly more textured meals and by the time she is one year old her food should be roughly mashed or very finely chopped. Give her three main meals a day, plus two or three healthy snacks between meals, such as a few finger foods or a small pot of fromage frais. At this age, children need to eat little and often as they are growing rapidly. This shouldn't affect their appetite at meal times, but obviously don't give snacks just before main meals and try not to give too many sweet sugary snacks such as biscuits (cookies).

You should still avoid seasoning food with salt, but you can start to use flavourings containing some salt, such as good-quality stock (bouillon) cubes, granules or powder. Some of the recipes here call for vegetable stock. You can use either the salt-free recipe on page 54 or commercially prepared stock.

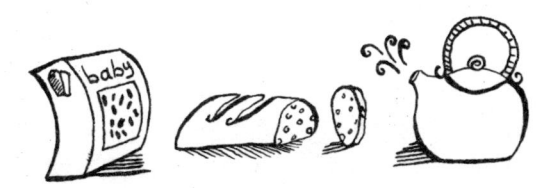

Finger foods

These not only provide useful nutrients but also aid your baby's co-ordination and help her on the way to self-feeding. Try to serve a selection, mixing high protein and carbohydrate foods with fresh fruit and vegetables. When she's teething, chewing and sucking will soothe sore gums and chilling sticks of raw fruit and vegetables before serving may help.

Simple ideas for finger foods

- Breadsticks, rusks, fingers of white or wholemeal (but not wholegrain) toast.
- Cooked pasta shapes.
- Cubes of cooked chicken.
- Cubes of mild cheese, such as Cheddar or Edam.
- Mini sandwiches.
- Pieces of dried sugar-free breakfast cereal (but not high-fibre varieties).
- Quartered, peeled and cored ripe pear or apple, peeled firm but ripe banana.
- Sticks of carrot or celery, cut into easy-to-hold pieces.

Foods to avoid at nine to twelve months

- ❖ Honey.
- ❖ Salt; but you can now use small amounts of stock, yeast extracts such as Marmite, and similar flavourings.
- ❖ Shellfish.
- ❖ Nuts, including peanut butter and sesame seeds.

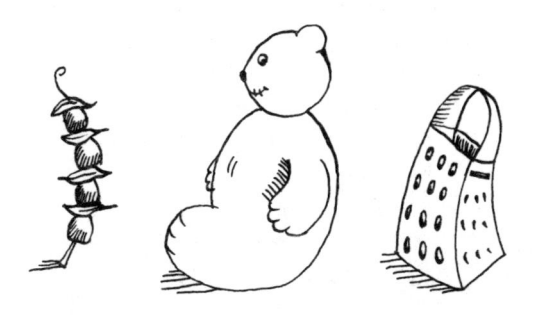

Chunky beef casserole

❋ MAKES 2 ADULT PLUS 2 BABY PORTIONS

350 g/12 oz braising steak
30 ml/2 tbsp sunflower oil
1 garlic clove, crushed
1 large onion, chopped
30 ml/2 tbsp plain (all-purpose) flour
600 ml/1 pint/2½ cups beef stock
5 ml/1 tsp soft light brown sugar
2.5 ml/½ tsp dried mixed herbs
10 ml/2 tsp Worcestershire sauce
15 ml/1 tbsp tomato purée (paste)
1 bay leaf
2 celery sticks, sliced
2 medium carrots, sliced
450 g/1 lb potatoes, peeled and cut into chunks
Salt and freshly ground blackpepper

1 Trim off any fat, then cut the meat into small cubes.

2 Heat 15 ml/1 tbsp of the oil in an ovenproof casserole dish (Dutch oven) and fry (sauté) the beef until well browned. Remove from the pan with a slotted spoon and set aside.

3. Heat the remaining oil in the casserole and gently fry the garlic and onion for 10 minutes. Sprinkle the flour over and stir in. Gradually stir in the stock, then the sugar, herbs, Worcestershire sauce and tomato purée. Add the bay leaf, celery and carrots.

4. Slowly bring to the boil, stirring until thickened. Cover and cook in a preheated oven at 160°C/325°F/gas 3/fan oven 145°C for 1½ hours.

5. Add the potatoes and cook for a further 30–40 minutes or until the meat and potatoes are tender.

6. Remove two baby portions. Season the remainder to be served as adult portions.

7. Chop the meat and vegetables for the baby portions, or purée until the desired consistency. Spoon half into a bowl and allow to cool slightly, if necessary, before serving.

8. Cool the remaining portion, cover and freeze, or store in the fridge for up to 24 hours.

Tip
If preferred, cook half the recipe quantity, purée to the desired consistency and divide into 10 baby-sized portions before freezing.

Beefy bean dinner

❋ MAKES 4 BABY PORTIONS

15 ml/1 tbsp sunflower oil
1 small onion, finely chopped
100 g/4 oz lean minced (ground) beef
50 g/2 oz macaroni
250 ml/8 fl oz/1 cup beef or vegetable stock (see page 54)
100 ml/3½ fl oz/scant ½ cup tomato juice
50 g/2 oz baked beans in tomato sauce

1. Heat the oil in a saucepan and gently fry (sauté) the onion for 5 minutes until beginning to soften. Add the minced beef and cook for a further 5 minutes until the meat is lightly browned.

2. Add the macaroni, stock and tomato juice. Stir once, cover and simmer for 15 minutes. Stir in the baked beans and cook for a further 5 minutes or until the pasta is tender.

3. Lightly chop or purée the mixture to the desired consistency. Spoon a portion into a bowl and allow to cool slightly, if necessary, before serving.

4. Cool the remaining mixture, divide into portions and freeze, or cover and store in the fridge for up to 24 hours.

Country pork with broccoli

❋ MAKES 4 BABY PORTIONS

100 g/4 oz lean pork, such as fillet
100 g/4 oz potatoes, roughly chopped
1 medium carrot, roughly chopped
300 ml/½ pint/1¼ cups vegetable stock (see page 54) or water
100 g/4 oz broccoli
60 ml/4 tbsp milk

1. Trim any fat from the pork and cut the meat into small cubes. Put the potatoes and carrot in a small saucepan with the stock or water. Bring to the boil, cover and simmer gently for 25 minutes.

2. Cut the broccoli into florets, add to the pan and cook for a further 10 minutes or until the meat and vegetables are tender. Remove from the heat, cool for a few minutes, then stir in the milk.

3. Purée the mixture to the desired consistency. Spoon a portion into a bowl and allow to cool slightly, if necessary, before serving.

4. Cool the remaining mixture, divide into portions and freeze, or cover and store in the fridge for up to 24 hours.

Shepherds' pie

❋ MAKES 2–3 ADULT PLUS 2 BABY PORTIONS

350 g/12 oz lean minced (ground) lamb
1 medium onion, finely chopped
50 g/2 oz mushrooms, finely chopped
2 carrots, finely diced
30 ml/2 tbsp plain (all-purpose) flour
300 ml/½ pint/1¼ cups lamb or vegetable stock (see page 54)
15 ml/1 tbsp tomato purée (paste)
1 bay leaf
Salt and freshly ground black pepper
700 g/1½ lb potatoes, cut into chunks
25 g/1 oz/2 tbsp butter or margarine
75 ml/5 tbsp milk

1 Fry (sauté) the minced lamb in a non-stick saucepan for 4–5 minutes until browned. Using a slotted spoon, transfer the meat to a plate, leaving the juices in the pan. Add the onion to the pan and cook gently for 10 minutes until softened and beginning to brown.

2 Add the mushrooms and carrots to the pan and fry for a further 2 minutes. Sprinkle the flour over and stir in. Gradually stir in the stock and tomato purée. Return the

3. Remove the bay leaf and spoon enough mixture to half-fill two 150 ml/¼ pint/⅔ cup ovenproof dishes. Season the remaining mixture with salt and pepper and spoon into a large ovenproof dish.

4. Meanwhile, cook the potatoes in boiling water for about 20 minutes until tender. Drain and mash with the butter or margarine and milk until smooth. Spoon a little over the meat mixture in the two small dishes. Season the remaining potato with salt and pepper and pile on to the meat mixture in the large dish.

5. Bake the pies in a preheated oven at 190°C/375°F/gas 5/fan oven 170°C, allowing 15 minutes for the small pies and 25 minutes for the larger one, until lightly browned.

6. Leave one of the baby portions to cool slightly before serving – this is quicker if you spoon it into a bowl. Cool the remaining portion completely. Cover and freeze, or store in the fridge for up to 24 hours.

Tip
If preferred, make up half the recipe quantity and use it to make eight baby portions.

Nine to Twelve Months

Bacon and bean feast

❋ MAKES 4 BABY PORTIONS

1 rasher (slice) of unsmoked back bacon
225 g/8 oz potatoes, cut into chunks
15 g/½ oz/1 tbsp butter or margarine
30 ml/2 tbsp milk
25 g/1 oz/¼ cup finely grated mild Cheddar cheese
200 g/7 oz /1 small can of baked beans in tomato sauce

1. Remove the fat and rind from the bacon. Chop the bacon into tiny pieces and dry-fry in a non-stick pan for 2–3 minutes until cooked.

2. Cook the potatoes in boiling water for 20 minutes or until tender. Drain well and mash with the butter or margarine, milk and cheese.

3. Lightly mash the beans with a fork, then add to the bacon and stir to mix. Divide the mixture between four 150 ml/ ¼ pint/⅔ cup ovenproof dishes and spoon the mashed potato on top.

4 Bake one of the portions in a preheated oven at 190°C/375°F/gas 5/fan oven 170°C for 20 minutes or until the top is golden brown. Alternatively, microwave on High for 5 minutes, then brown the top under a grill (broiler) for 1 minute, if liked. Leave to cool to the desired serving temperature.

5 Cover and freeze the remaining portions, or store in the fridge for up to 24 hours.

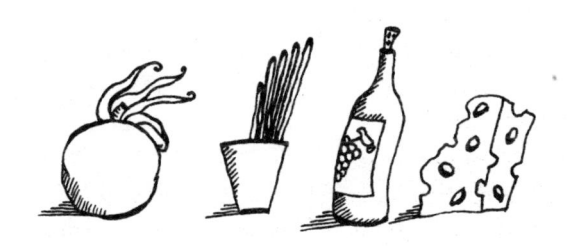

Fruity lamb couscous

❇ MAKES 4 BABY PORTIONS

50 g/2 oz/⅓ cup mixed dried fruit, such as apple rings, apricots and prunes
300 ml/½ pint/1¼ cups lamb or vegetable stock (see page 54)
175 g/6 oz lean lamb, such as fillet
10 ml/2 tsp sunflower oil
1 medium carrot, finely chopped
5 ml/1 tsp tomato purée (paste)
50 g/2 oz/⅓ cup couscous

1 Rinse the fruit under cold running water to remove any preservatives. Chop finely and put in a bowl. Pour over the stock or water and leave to soak for at least 1 hour.

2 Trim any fat from the lamb and cut it into small cubes. Heat the oil in a saucepan and fry (sauté) the lamb until browned. Add the carrot and cook for 1 minute, stirring all the time.

3 Stir in the fruit with the stock or water and tomato purée. Cover and simmer gently for 30 minutes or until the lamb is almost tender.

4 Put the couscous in a sieve (strainer) and rinse under cold running water. Place the sieve over the lamb in the pan, cover and steam for 20 minutes.

5 Chop or process the lamb and vegetable mixture to the desired consistency. Stir in the steamed couscous.

6 Spoon a portion into a bowl and allow to cool slightly, if necessary, before serving.

7 Cool the remainder, divide into portions and freeze, or cover and store in the fridge for up to 24 hours.

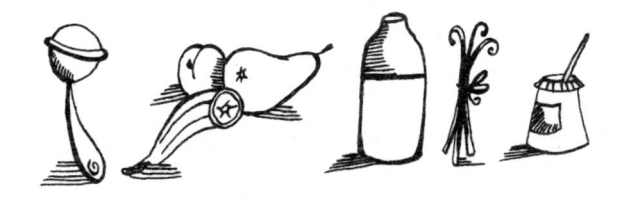

Paprika pork with rice and beans

❊ MAKES 4 BABY PORTIONS

100 g/4 oz lean pork, such as fillet
10 ml/2 tsp sunflower oil
50 g/2 oz/¼ cup long-grain rice
1.5 ml/¼ tsp paprika
300 ml/½ pint/1¼ cups milk
75 g/3 oz/½ cup baked beans in tomato sauce

1. Cut the pork into 5 mm/¼ in cubes. Heat the oil in a non-stick saucepan and cook the pork until lightly browned. Stir in the rice and paprika, then pour in the milk. Bring to the boil and simmer, uncovered, for 12 minutes.

2. Stir in the beans, lower the heat, cover and cook for a further 2–3 minutes or until the pork and rice are tender. Lightly mash or purée to the desired consistency.

3. Spoon a portion into a bowl and allow to cool slightly, if necessary, before serving.

4. Cool the remainder, divide into portions and freeze, or cover and store in the fridge for up to 24 hours.

Lamb and lentil supper

❋ MAKES 4 BABY PORTIONS

100 g/4 oz lean lamb, such as fillet
25 g/1 oz/2 tbsp red lentils
100 g/4 oz sweet potato, cut into chunks
5 ml/1 tsp tomato purée (paste)
350 ml/12 fl oz/1⅓ cups lamb or vegetable stock (see page 54)

1 Trim any fat from the lamb and cut it into small cubes. Put the lentils in a sieve (strainer) and rinse under cold water.

2 Put all the ingredients in a small saucepan. Slowly bring to the boil, cover and simmer gently for 35 minutes or until the lamb and lentils are tender. Check towards the end of the cooking time and add a little more stock or water if needed.

3 Mash or purée the mixture to the desired consistency. Spoon a portion into a bowl and allow to cool slightly, if necessary, before serving.

4 Cool the remaining mixture, divide into portions and freeze, or cover and store in the fridge for up to 24 hours.

Turkey and tomato hotpot

❋ MAKES 4 BABY PORTIONS

100 g/4 oz turkey breast, skinned and boned
50 g/2 oz/¼ cup long-grain rice
150 ml/¼ pint/⅔ cup chicken or turkey stock
150 ml/¼ pint/⅔ cup tomato juice
25 g/1 oz frozen peas

1. Cut the turkey into thin strips. Put in a small saucepan with all the remaining ingredients. Bring to the boil, cover and simmer for 15 minutes or until the turkey and rice are cooked.

2. Purée the mixture to the desired consistency. Spoon a portion into a bowl and allow to cool slightly, if necessary, before serving.

3. Cool the remaining mixture, divide into portions and freeze, or cover and store in the fridge for up to 24 hours.

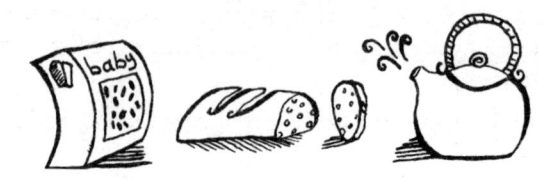

Chicken and vegetable bites

MAKES 1 BABY PORTION

1 medium carrot
100 g/4 oz potato
50 g/2 oz cooked chicken
15 ml/1 tbsp canned or frozen sweetcorn (corn), thawed
1 egg yolk
15 ml/1 tbsp plain (all-purpose) flour
30 ml/2 tbsp sunflower oil

1 Peel the carrot and potato and grate them coarsely. Squeeze out as much liquid as possible, then pat dry with kitchen paper (paper towels). Put in a bowl.

2 Finely chop the chicken. Add to the grated vegetables with the sweetcorn and egg yolk. Mix well. Sprinkle the flour over and mix again.

3 Heat the oil in a large frying pan (skillet) over a medium heat. Drop spoonfuls of the mixture into the pan, lightly pressing down with the back of the spoon to flatten. Cook for about 3 minutes on each side until lightly browned and cooked through.

4 Drain on kitchen paper and allow to cool for a few minutes before serving.

Fisherman's pie

❋ MAKES 2 ADULT PLUS 2 BABY PORTIONS

225 g/8 oz cod or haddock fillet
300 ml/½ pint/1¼ cups milk
1 bay leaf
1 small onion, sliced
40 g/1½ oz/3 tbsp butter or margarine
30 ml/2 tbsp plain (all-purpose) flour
1 egg, hard-boiled (hard-cooked) and finely chopped
15 ml/1 tbsp chopped fresh parsley
Salt and freshly ground black pepper
225 g/8 oz potatoes, cut into chunks
100 g/4 oz carrots, cut into chunks
30 ml/2 tbsp plain Greek yoghurt

1. Put the fish in a pan with the milk, bay leaf and onion. Slowly bring to boiling point, then simmer gently for 6 minutes or until the fish is opaque. Lift the fish from the pan using a slotted spoon and remove the skin and bones. Strain the milk and reserve.

2. Melt 25 g/1 oz/2 tbsp of the butter or margarine in a pan. Stir in the flour and cook gently for 1 minute. Remove from the heat and gradually stir in the reserved milk. Bring to the boil and simmer for 2–3 minutes until thickened.

3 Stir the fish, egg and parsley into the sauce. Half-fill two 150 ml/¼ pint/⅔ cup ovenproof dishes with the fish mixture. Season the remainder with salt and pepper and spoon into an ovenproof pie dish.

4 Cook the potatoes and carrots in boiling water for 20 minutes until tender. Drain well and mash with the remaining butter or margarine and the yoghurt. Spoon a little over the fish mixture in the individual dishes, then season the rest and use to top the fish in the pie dish.

5 Bake the baby portions in a preheated oven at 200°C/400°F/gas 6/fan oven 180°C for 15 minutes and the adults' pie for 20–25 minutes or until the tops are lightly browned.

6 Allow one of the baby portions to cool to the temperature desired before serving.

7 Cool the remaining portion, cover and freeze, or store in the fridge for up to 24 hours.

Tip
If preferred, cook half the recipe quantity and divide it into eight baby-sized portions before freezing.

Cheesy cod and broccoli

❊ MAKES 4 BABY PORTIONS

100 g/4 oz broccoli
225 g/8 oz potatoes, diced
100 g/4 oz frozen skinless cod
300 ml/½ pint/1¼ cups milk
50 g/2 oz/½ cup grated mild Cheddar cheese

1. Cut the broccoli into florets. Put it in a saucepan with the potatoes, cod and milk.

2. Bring to the boil and simmer gently, uncovered, for 15 minutes or until the fish is cooked and the vegetables are tender. Remove from the heat, add the cheese and stir until melted.

3. Mash the mixture to the desired consistency. Spoon a portion into a bowl and allow to cool slightly, if necessary, before serving.

4. Cool the remaining purée, divide into portions and freeze, or cover and store in the fridge for up to 24 hours.

Butter baked salmon with dill

❋ MAKES 4 BABY PORTIONS

100 g/4 oz salmon fillet
5 ml/1 tsp lemon juice
25 g/1 oz/2 tbsp butter or margarine
15 ml/1 tbsp plain (all-purpose) flour
120 ml/4 fl oz/½ cup milk
15 ml/1 tbsp finely chopped fresh dill (dill weed)

1 Put the salmon on a piece of foil, sprinkle with the lemon juice and top with half the butter or margarine. Bake in a preheated oven at 180°C/350°F/gas 4/fan oven 160°C for 15 minutes or until cooked through.

2 Meanwhile, put the remaining butter or margarine, the flour and milk in a small pan. Slowly bring to the boil, whisking all the time, until smooth and thick. Simmer for 1 minute.

3 Strain the juices from the fish into the sauce. Flake the fish, then lightly mash with a fork, removing any skin and bones. Stir into the sauce with the dill.

4 Spoon a portion into a bowl and allow to cool slightly, if necessary, before serving.

5 Cool the remainder, divide into portions and freeze, or cover and store in the fridge for up to 24 hours.

Creamy carrot mousse

This light, baked savoury mousse makes a tasty vegetable accompaniment for adult meals too.

❋ MAKES 4 BABY PORTIONS

275 g/10 oz carrots, roughly chopped
1 small red (bell) pepper, halved, seeded and chopped
45 ml/3 tbsp vegetable stock (see page 54) or water
2 eggs
100 g/4 oz/½ cup plain fromage frais

1 Lightly grease four 150 ml/¼ pint/⅔ cup ramekins (custard cups) or small pudding basins and line the bases with greaseproof (waxed) paper.

2 Put the chopped vegetables in a small saucepan with the stock or water. Cover and cook gently for 10 minutes or until very soft. Remove the lid for the last 2–3 minutes to allow the liquid to evaporate.

3 Sieve (strain) or purée the mixture in a food processor until fairly smooth.

4 Lightly whisk the eggs and fromage frais together. Stir in the vegetable purée. Divide the mixture between the prepared dishes, then cover each one with a piece of greased foil.

5. Put the dishes in a roasting tin (pan) and pour enough hot water into the tin to come about half way up the dishes. Bake in a preheated oven at 180°C/350°F/gas 4/fan oven 160°C for 40 minutes or until lightly set.

6. Turn out one of the mousses into a bowl and allow to cool slightly, if necessary, before serving.

7. Cool the remaining mousses and freeze, or cover and store in the fridge for up to 24 hours.

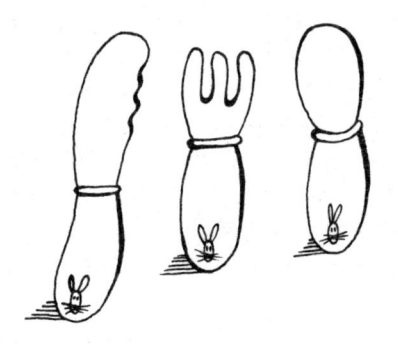

Nine to Twelve Months

Pasta with mushroom sauce

MAKES 1 BABY PORTION

1 ripe tomato
3 button mushrooms, finely chopped
15 g/½ oz/1 tbsp butter or margarine
15 ml/1 tbsp Mascarpone cheese
30 ml/2 tbsp milk
15 g/½ oz mini pasta shapes

1 Plunge the tomato into boiling water and leave for 1 minute. Remove, peel off the skin, halve, seed and finely chop. Wipe and chop the mushrooms.

2 Melt the butter or margarine in a small saucepan. Add the mushrooms and cook gently for 3 minutes, then add the tomato and cook for a further 2–3 minutes or until very soft. Stir in the cheese and milk and heat until melted.

3 Meanwhile, cook the pasta in boiling water for 6 minutes until tender, or according to the packet instructions. Drain well.

4 Stir the pasta into the mushroom sauce and spoon into a bowl. Allow to cool slightly, if necessary, before serving.

Tip
You can buy tiny pasta shapes, usually labelled 'mini' or 'soup' pasta, such as farfalline, which are ideal baby food as they don't need to be chewed.

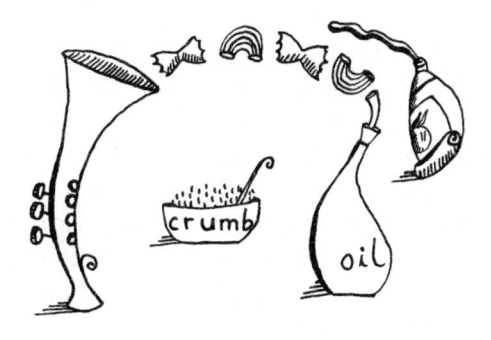

Main meal minestrone

MAKES 2 ADULT PLUS 1 BABY PORTION

15 ml/1 tbsp olive oil
2 rashers (slices) of streaky bacon, rinded and chopped
1 large onion, chopped
1 garlic clove, crushed
2 medium carrots, finely diced
2 celery sticks, diced
1 medium potato, diced
A pinch of dried oregano
45 ml/3 tbsp red wine (optional)
200 g/7 oz/1 small can of chopped tomatoes
600 ml/1 pint/2½ cups chicken stock
40 g/1½ oz short-cut macaroni
100 g/4 oz/1 cup cooked chicken, skinned and finely chopped
Salt and freshly ground black pepper
To serve:
Freshly grated Parmesan cheese

1 Heat the oil in a flameproof casserole dish (Dutch oven) or saucepan. Add the bacon and cook for a few minutes until crisp. Remove from the pan with a slotted spoon and set aside.

2. Add the onion and garlic to the pan and gently fry (sauté) for 10 minutes until soft. Stir in the carrots, celery and potato and cook for a further 5 minutes, stirring all the time. Add the oregano, the wine, if using, and the tomatoes and stock.

3. Bring to the boil, turn down the heat, cover and simmer for 25 minutes.

4. Add the macaroni to the pan and simmer, uncovered, for 8 minutes. Stir in the chicken and bacon and simmer for a further 2–3 minutes or until the pasta is tender.

5. Remove a portion of the minestrone for baby. Lightly mash with a fork, then allow it to cool slightly, if necessary, before serving.

6. Season the adult portions with salt and pepper and serve with freshly grated Parmesan cheese.

Tip
It's perfectly all right to add a little wine to a recipe like this, as all the alcohol evaporates during cooking.

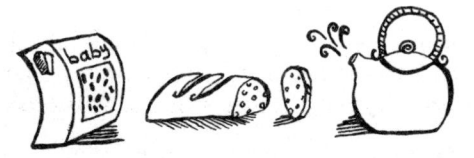

Pasta primavera

❋ MAKES 4 BABY PORTIONS

2 ripe tomatoes
1 medium carrot, diced
1 small courgette (zucchini), diced
25 g/1 oz green (French) beans, diced
250 ml/8 fl oz/1 cup milk
40 g/1½ oz mini pasta shapes
25 g/1 oz/¼ cup finely grated mild Cheddar cheese

1 Plunge the tomatoes into boiling water. Leave for 1 minute, then remove and peel. Halve, seed and cut into tiny dice.

2 Put the carrot, courgette and beans in a pan with the milk. Bring to the boil, part-cover with a lid and simmer for 10 minutes.

3 Add the tomatoes and pasta. Stir once, then simmer, uncovered, for a further 5 minutes until the pasta and vegetables are cooked. Remove from the heat, add the cheese and stir until melted.

4 Spoon a portion into a bowl and allow to cool slightly, if necessary, before serving.

5 Cool the remaining mixture, divide into portions and freeze, or cover and store in the fridge for up to 24 hours.

Spaghetti junction

❋ MAKES 4 BABY PORTIONS

250 ml/8 fl oz/1 cup milk
50 g/2 oz fine quick-cook spaghetti
25 g/1 oz frozen mixed vegetables
50 g/2 oz wafer-thin slices of roast ham, finely chopped

1. Bring the milk to the boil in a small saucepan. Break the spaghetti into short lengths, add to the milk and simmer, uncovered, for 4 minutes.

2. Add the vegetables, part-cover with a lid and simmer for a further 5 minutes or until the spaghetti and vegetables are tender. Remove from the heat. Stir in the ham.

3. Lightly mash with a fork or purée to the desired consistency. Spoon a portion into a bowl and allow to cool slightly, if necessary, before serving.

4. Cool the remaining mixture, divide into portions and freeze, or cover and store in the fridge for up to 24 hours.

Tip
The spaghetti will absorb the milk as it cools and you may have to add a little extra milk when reheating from frozen.

Savoury spinach custard

MAKES 1 BABY PORTION

50 g/2 oz frozen spinach, thawed
15 g/½ oz/1 tbsp butter or margarine
1 egg
75 ml/5 tbsp milk

1. Thoroughly drain the spinach. Chop finely and put in a small pan with the butter or margarine. Cook gently for 3 minutes until fairly dry. Remove from the heat and allow to cool for a few minutes.

2. Whisk together the egg and milk. Stir into the spinach, then spoon the mixture into a greased 150 ml/¼ pint/⅔ cup ramekin (custard cup).

3. Bake in a preheated oven at 160°C/325°F/gas 3/fan oven 145°C for 30 minutes or until set. Allow to cool slightly before serving.

Tip
This recipe is ideal for using up leftover vegetables, such as diced carrot or chopped cauliflower or broccoli, instead of the spinach.

Cream cheese and ham pasta

MAKES 1 BABY PORTION

1 wafer-thin slice of honey roast ham
15 g/½ oz mini pasta shapes
15 g/½ oz/1 tbsp cream cheese
15 ml/1 tbsp milk

1 Finely chop the ham. Cook the pasta in a small saucepan of boiling water for 5 minutes or until tender. Drain well.

2 Heat the cream cheese and the milk in the pan, stirring until it melts to a sauce. Stir in the pasta and ham. Serve as soon as it has cooled enough to eat.

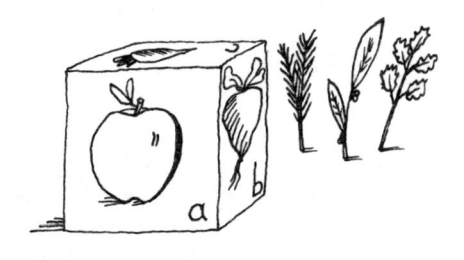

French toast fingers

MAKES 1 BABY PORTION

1 slice of bread
½ egg, beaten
15 ml/1 tbsp milk
15 g/½ oz/1 tbsp butter or margarine
15 ml/1 tbsp sunflower oil

1. Trim the crusts off the bread. Whisk the egg and milk together, then dip in the bread, turning after a few seconds to coat both sides.

2. Heat the butter or margarine and oil in a frying pan (skillet) until sizzling. Add the bread and cook for about 1½ minutes on each side or until golden brown.

3. Cool slightly, then cut into four strips. Serve as a meal or as finger food.

Tip
Put any remaining beaten egg in a small bowl, cover and store in the fridge for up to 24 hours.

Chocolate drop pudding

MAKES 1 BABY PORTION

15 ml/1 tbsp ground rice
5 ml/1 tsp caster (superfine) sugar
120 ml/4 fl oz/½ cup milk
25 g/1 oz/¼ cup milk chocolate drops

1 Put the rice and sugar in a small saucepan and gradually blend in the milk. Bring to the boil and simmer gently for 10–12 minutes, stirring occasionally, until the mixture has thickened and the rice is cooked. Remove from the heat and allow to cool for a few minutes.

2 Stir in the chocolate drops while the rice is still warm, then spoon into a bowl. Serve as the chocolate begins to melt.

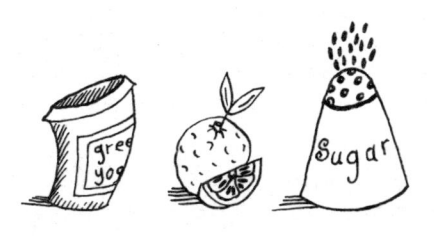

Vanilla creams

MAKES 2 BABY PORTIONS

10 ml/2 tsp caster (superfine) sugar
2.5 ml/½ tsp cornflour (cornstarch)
1.5 ml/¼ tsp vanilla essence (extract)
1 egg
150 ml/¼ pint/⅔ cup milk

1. Whisk the sugar, cornflour, vanilla essence and egg together in a jug. Pour the milk into a saucepan and heat to boiling point. Pour the milk over the egg mixture, whisking all the time.

2. Divide the mixture between two lightly greased ramekins (custard cups) and place in a roasting tin (pan). Pour enough warm water into the tin to come about half way up the ramekins.

3. Bake in a preheated oven at 180°C/350°F/gas 4/fan oven 160°C for 20 minutes or until just set. Remove from the water and leave to cool. Serve one portion at room temperature.

4. Cover and chill the remaining vanilla cream. Serve cold within 24 hours. Do not reheat.

Fresh fruity jelly

MAKES 2 OR 3 BABY PORTIONS

300 ml/½ pint/1¼ cups fresh fruit juice, such as orange
10 ml/2 tsp powdered gelatine

1. Spoon 60 ml/4 tbsp of the fruit juice into a small bowl. Sprinkle the gelatine over and leave to soak for 5 minutes. Place the bowl over a pan of near-boiling water until the gelatine has dissolved, stirring occasionally. Cool for a few minutes, then stir the dissolved gelatine into the rest of the juice.

2. Divide between two or three individual dishes. Chill in the fridge for at least 3 hours, or overnight, until set.

3. Remove one portion from the fridge about 20 minutes before serving to take the chill off.

4. Cover the remaining portion(s) and store in the fridge for up to 48 hours.

Tip
Use any of your baby's favourite fruit juices, such as apple, peach or tropical fruit. If liked, make a Fruit and Fromage Frais Jelly by substituting 150 ml/¼ pint/⅔ cup of the fruit juice with plain or fruit-flavoured fromage frais. Serve within 24 hours of making.

Chocolate milk jelly

MAKES 2 BABY PORTIONS

200 ml/7 fl oz/scant 1 cup milk
5 ml/1 tsp powdered gelatine
5 ml/1 tsp cocoa (unsweetened chocolate) powder
5 ml/1 tsp caster (superfine) sugar

1. Spoon 30 ml/2 tbsp of the milk into a small bowl and sprinkle the gelatine over. Leave to soak for 5 minutes. Place over a pan of near-boiling water until dissolved, stirring occasionally.

2. Meanwhile, blend the cocoa powder and sugar with a little of the remaining milk in a small saucepan. Whisk in all of the remaining milk and bring to the boil. Remove from the heat.

3. Add the soaked gelatine to the chocolate milk and stir until dissolved. Pour into two small dishes or jelly moulds. Allow to cool, then put in the fridge to set.

4. Remove one portion from the fridge about 20 minutes before serving to take the chill off.

5. Cover the remaining portion and serve within 24 hours.

Tip
The jelly can be served in the dishes or turned out if preferred. Dip the dishes in very hot water for a few seconds to loosen, place a plate or bowl on top of the dish and invert.

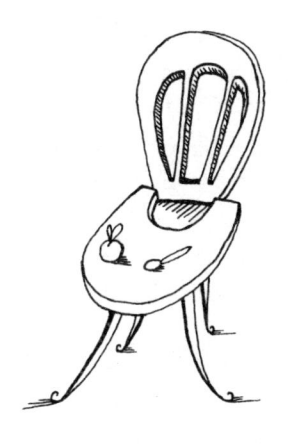

Steamed banana custard

MAKES 1 BABY PORTION

½ ripe banana
1 egg
45 ml/3 tbsp milk
2.5 ml/½ tsp caster (superfine) sugar
A few drops of vanilla essence (extract)

1 Peel and thinly slice the banana and place in a greased 150 ml/¼ pint/⅔ cup ramekin (custard cup).

2 Whisk the egg, milk, sugar and vanilla essence together. Pour over the banana slices. Cover with a piece of foil and place in a steamer.

3 Cover and steam over gently boiling water for about 15 minutes, until set. Allow to cool slightly before serving.

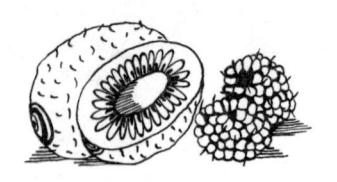

Apricot fool

❋ MAKES 4 BABY PORTIONS

100 g/4 oz/⅔ cup dried apricots
150 ml/¼ pint/⅔ cup apple or peach juice
To serve:
Plain Greek yoghurt

1. Rinse the apricots under cold running water to remove any preservatives. Chop finely and put in a small saucepan with the apple or peach juice. Leave to soak for at least 2 hours.

2. Cook over a gentle heat for 4–5 minutes or until the apricots are very soft. Purée until smooth. Leave to cool.

3. Spoon a quarter of the apricot purée into a bowl and stir in 15 ml/1 tbsp of Greek yoghurt.

4. Divide the remaining purée into portions and freeze, or cover and store in the fridge for up to 24 hours.

Tip
Freeze the apricot purée without the yoghurt.

From Baby to Toddler

Your child is now nearing the stage when she will eat more or less the same sort of food as the rest of the family and there's no longer any need to purée her meals. Encourage her to become familiar with a wide variety of foods. You may wish to give 'follow-on' milk for a few more months, or to switch to full-fat cows' milk; skimmed and semi-skimmed milk and low-fat foods should be avoided until the age of two, as they don't have the concentration of calories needed by young children and have less of the vitamins A and D. Try to cook healthily though, by trimming fat from meat and cooking with vegetable rather than saturated animal fats. You should also avoid too many meals of fried (sautéed) food, processed meat like salami, sausages and pies and frequent high-fat snacks such as crisps (chips) and chocolate. You'll find a selection of desserts and bakes in this chapter; serve them as occasional treats rather than daily – fresh and dried fruit, yoghurt and fromage frais are all easy and healthy alternatives.

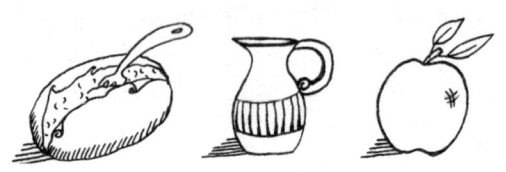

Fussy eaters

Nearly all children are fickle eaters at times and quickly learn to assert themselves and to let you know what they do and don't like. They may have a fad which goes on for days or even weeks and the lovingly prepared food they enjoyed yesterday may be rejected today. This can be very trying for you, but try to respect your baby's individuality, within reason, and to find alternatives to the foods that are refused. If milk is turned down, offer yoghurt or flavoured milk jelly; if she's eating plenty of fruit, it really doesn't matter if she leaves all her vegetables. Think of food intake on a weekly rather than a daily basis; hopefully if your child rejects a meal one day, she'll make up for it the next. A balanced diet over several weeks is perfectly acceptable. If your child refuses a meal (assuming you haven't given her something you know she doesn't like), don't rush away and prepare an alternative or offer sweets and biscuits later or she'll soon discover that this is a good ploy to get what she wants. If you're worried that your child is really hungry, bring the next meal time forward. If that's not convenient, offer some toast or bread and butter or margarine. If your toddler is going through a 'picky' phase, don't spend hours in the kitchen preparing meals; choose something quick and easy, or you'll end up even more frustrated when she refuses to eat. Try to accept that toddlers' appetites are unpredictable and there will inevitably be days when they eat practically nothing.

From Baby to Toddler

Children often dislike the texture of meat. Try finely minced (ground) meats instead, but if your child refuses these as well, don't worry, as there are plenty of other good sources of protein, such as dairy produce and eggs. Protein is also found in reasonable quantities in pulses (beans and lentils), peanut butter and bread.

Encourage an interest in food by making it look as attractive as possible. Try arranging it in patterns or make it look like a face, if you have the time and patience. Otherwise, adding eyes, nose and a smiling mouth in ketchup (catsup) sometimes works wonders!

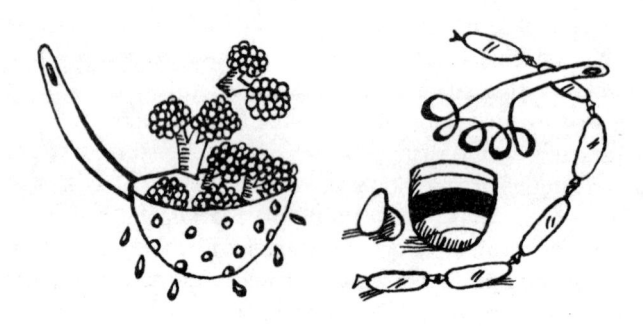

Crunchy chicken nuggets

❋ MAKES 6 BABY PORTIONS

225 g/8 oz skinless chicken breast
50 g/2 oz/1 cup fresh white breadcrumbs
100 g/4 oz/1 cup cooked long-grain rice
1 egg, beaten
15 ml/1 tbsp chopped fresh parsley (optional)
Salt and freshly ground black pepper
25 g/1 oz/¼ cup plain (all-purpose) flour
30 ml/2 tbsp sunflower oil

1. Roughly chop the chicken and process in a food processor until just smooth. Alternatively, chop very finely.

2. Transfer the chicken to a bowl. Add the breadcrumbs, rice, egg and parsley, if using. Lightly season with salt and pepper and mix well.

3. Using floured hands, shape into 18 equal-sized balls and place on a baking (cookie) sheet.

4. Heat the oil in a frying pan (skillet) and cook three of the chicken nuggets for 6 minutes, turning until browned all over and cooked through. Allow to cool slightly before serving.

5. Open-freeze the remaining nuggets, then pack in portions in freezerproof containers or bags.

Easy cheese and tomato pizza puffs

MAKES 2 ADULT PLUS 1 BABY PORTION

350 g/12 oz puff pastry (paste)
45 ml/3 tbsp sun-dried tomato purée (paste)
30 ml/2 tbsp Mascarpone cheese
A pinch of dried mixed herbs
75 g/3 oz/¾ cup finely grated Cheddar cheese
15 cherry tomatoes, halved

1 Roll out the pastry on a lightly floured work surface and cut out five 13 cm/5 in rounds using a small plate or saucer as a guide. Transfer to a lightly greased baking (cookie) sheet and prick all over with a fork. Chill in the fridge for 20 minutes.

2 Mix together the tomato purée, Mascarpone and herbs. Spread evenly over the pastry bases. Sprinkle half the Cheddar over the top, then arrange the cherry tomatoes over it, cut-sides up. Sprinkle with the remaining Cheddar.

3 Bake on the middle shelf in a preheated oven at 220°C/425°F/gas 7/fan oven 200°C for 14–15 minutes or until the pastry is golden and crisp and the cheese lightly browned and bubbling.

4. Allow to cool on the baking sheet for a few minutes – the cheese and tomatoes will be very hot. Serve two pizza puffs for each adult and one for baby.

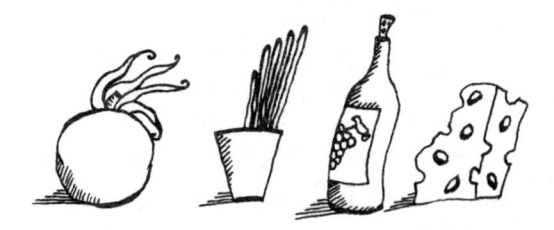

Creamy chicken korma

This very mild curry is a great introduction to spicy foods and you can jazz up the adults' servings with some hot Indian pickles.

MAKES 2 ADULT PLUS 1 BABY PORTION

15 ml/1 tbsp ghee or sunflower oil
1 large onion, finely chopped
1 garlic clove, crushed
5 ml/1 tsp ground coriander (cilantro)
1.5 ml/¼ tsp ground ginger
1.5 ml/¼ tsp ground cumin
2 boneless chicken breasts, skinned
5 ml/1 tsp lemon juice
400 ml/14 fl oz/1¾ cups thick plain yoghurt
75 ml/5 tbsp chicken or vegetable stock (see page 54)
Salt and freshly ground black pepper
To serve:
Rice or naan bread

1. Heat the ghee or oil in a saucepan and gently fry (sauté) the onion for 5 minutes. Add the garlic and cook for a further 5 minutes or until the onion is soft and just beginning to colour. Stir in the spices and cook, stirring all the time, for 1 minute.

2. Meanwhile, cut each chicken breast into four pieces. Add to the pan with the lemon juice. Turn the heat down as low as possible, then stir in three-quarters of the yoghurt, a spoonful at a time.

3. Stir in the stock. Part-cover the pan with a lid and simmer gently for about 30 minutes until the chicken is very tender and cooked through.

4. Remove one or two pieces of chicken for baby and chop very finely. Put in a bowl and mix with a spoonful of the sauce and a little extra yoghurt. Stir in a spoonful of rice or serve with strips of warmed naan bread.

5. Season the remaining korma with salt and pepper and serve to the adults topped with a drizzle of yoghurt and some hot pickles and rice or naan bread.

Tip
Choose Bio or Greek-style yoghurt for this recipe as it has a creamier, less tangy flavour than ordinary yoghurt.

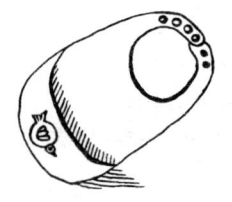

Crumble-topped lamb casserole

MAKES 2 ADULT PLUS 1 BABY PORTION

350 g/12 oz lean lamb, such as boned leg or shoulder
30 ml/2 tbsp sunflower oil
1 onion, finely chopped
15 ml/1 tbsp plain (all-purpose) flour
150 ml/¼ pint/⅔ cup lamb or vegetable stock (see page 54)
175 g/6 oz carrots, diced
175 g/6 oz turnips, diced
200 g/7 oz/1 small can of chopped tomatoes
2.5 ml/½ tsp dried thyme
1 bay leaf
Salt and freshly ground black pepper
For the topping:
100 g/4 oz/1 cup plain (all-purpose) flour
50 g/2 oz/¼ cup butter or margarine
50 g/2 oz/½ cup finely grated Cheddar cheese

1 Trim any fat from the lamb and cut into tiny cubes. Heat the oil in a 1.75 litre/3 pint/7½ cup flameproof casserole (Dutch oven) and fry (sauté) the lamb until lightly browned. Remove from the casserole with a slotted spoon.

2 Add the onion to the casserole and fry for 5 minutes, until beginning to soften and brown. Sprinkle the flour over and stir in. Gradually add the stock, then stir in the carrots, turnips, tomatoes, herbs and a little seasoning.

3 Bring to the boil, stirring occasionally. Cover and cook in a preheated oven at 160°C/325°F/gas 3/fan oven 145°C for 1 hour.

4 Meanwhile, make the topping. Sift the flour into a bowl. Cut the butter or margarine into small cubes and rub in until the mixture resembles breadcrumbs. Stir in the grated cheese.

5 Turn up the oven to 180°C/350°F/gas 5/fan oven 160°C. Sprinkle the topping over the casserole, return to the oven and cook, uncovered, for a further 30–35 minutes or until lightly browned. Cool the baby portion before serving.

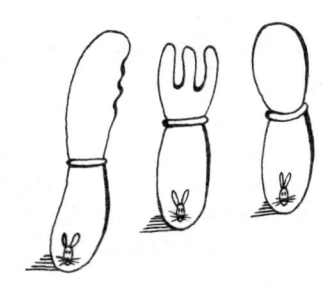

From Baby to Toddler

Chicken satay sticks

These tasty chicken skewers make ideal finger food, but remember to remove the meat from the skewers and take them away before serving. Do read the section on allergies on page 21 before giving peanut butter to your baby.

MAKES 2 ADULT PLUS 1 BABY PORTION

350 g/12 oz skinless chicken breast
10 ml/2 tsp sesame oil
15 ml/1 tbsp sunflower oil
10 ml/2 tsp lemon juice
10 ml/2 tsp soy sauce
15 ml/1 tbsp clear honey
For the peanut dip:
25 g/1 oz creamed coconut
75 ml/5 tbsp water
A small pinch of mild chilli powder
50 g/2 oz/4 tbsp smooth peanut butter
10 ml/2 tsp dark soft brown sugar
5 ml/1 tsp lemon juice

1 Cut the chicken into cubes. Mix together the oils, lemon juice, soy sauce and honey. Add the chicken, toss to coat, then cover and marinate in the fridge for 2 hours.

From Baby to Toddler

2 Meanwhile, make the peanut dip. Roughly chop the creamed coconut and put in a small pan with the water. Heat gently until melted. Stir in the chilli powder, peanut butter, sugar and lemon juice. Stir until combined, then spoon into a serving bowl.

3 Thread the chicken on to skewers. Cook under a hot grill (broiler) for 8–10 minutes, turning occasionally and brushing with the marinade, until cooked through.

4 Serve the chicken satay warm or cold with the peanut dip.

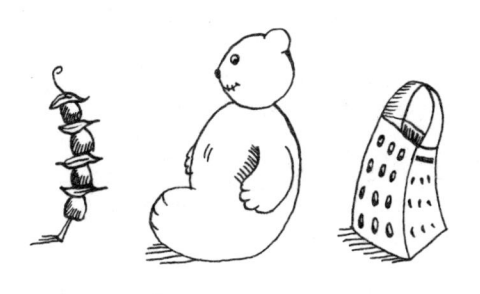

Lamb and lentil lasagne

MAKES 2 ADULT PLUS 1 BABY PORTION

15 ml/1 tbsp olive oil
1 onion, finely chopped
225 g/8 oz lean minced (ground) lamb
2.5 ml/½ tsp dried oregano
40 g/1½ oz/⅓ cup plain (all-purpose) flour
150 ml/¼ pint/⅔ cup lamb or vegetable stock (see page 54)
15 ml/1 tbsp tomato purée (paste)
25 g/1 oz/2 tbsp red lentils
Salt and freshly ground black pepper
25 g/1 oz/2 tbsp butter or margarine
300 ml/½ pint/1¼ cups milk
75 g/3 oz/¾ cup finely grated Cheddar cheese
6 no-need-to-precook lasagne sheets

1 Heat the oil in a saucepan and gently cook the onion for 10 minutes until soft and just beginning to brown. Remove from the pan and set aside.

2. Add the lamb to the pan and cook until browned. Pour off any excess fat. Return the onion to the pan with the oregano. Sprinkle over 15 ml/1 tbsp of the flour and stir in. Gradually add the stock, tomato purée, lentils and a little salt and pepper. Cover and simmer for 20 minutes.

3. Meanwhile, put the remaining flour, the butter or margarine and milk in a saucepan and slowly bring to the boil, stirring all the time until thickened and smooth. Remove from the heat and stir in 50 g/2 oz/½ cup of the cheese.

4. Layer the lamb mixture alternately with the lasagne sheets in a lightly greased, deep, ovenproof serving dish. Spoon over the cheese sauce, then sprinkle with the remaining cheese.

5. Bake in a preheated oven at 190°C/375°F/gas 5/fan oven 170°C for 35 minutes or until the lasagne is cooked and the topping brown and bubbling.

6. Spoon the baby portion into a bowl and chop the lasagne into small pieces. Allow to cool to the desired temperature before serving.

From Baby to Toddler

Crunchy fish fingers

Do read the section on allergies on page 21 before giving sesame seeds to your baby.

❈ MAKES 3 BABY PORTIONS

350 g/12 oz plaice fillets
30 ml/2 tbsp plain (all-purpose) flour
1 egg
75 g/3 oz/1½ cups fresh white breadcrumbs
15 ml/1 tbsp sesame seeds
To serve:
Mashed potatoes or chips (fries) and a green vegetable

1. Skin the plaice, rinse under cold water and pat dry on kitchen paper (paper towels). Cut into thin strips and toss in the flour to coat.

2. Lightly beat the egg. Mix together the breadcrumbs and sesame seeds and place on a plate. Dip the floured fish strips, one at a time, in the egg, then in the breadcrumbs. Place a third of the fish fingers on a lightly greased baking (cookie) sheet.

3 Bake in a preheated oven at 200°C/400°F/gas 6/fan oven 180°C for about 12 minutes or until crisp and golden brown. Serve straight away with mashed potatoes or chips and a green vegetable.

4 Put the remaining fish fingers on a baking sheet and open-freeze until solid. Remove from the tray, place in a freezerproof container or bag and freeze until required.

Tip
Make sure that you buy fresh plaice fillets that have not been previously frozen.

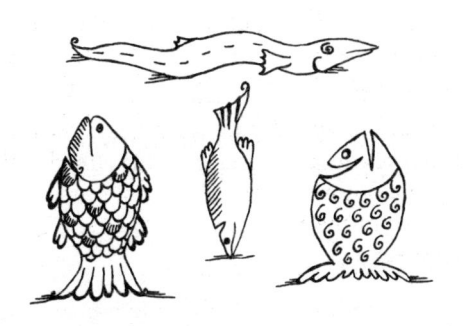

Chicken goujons with chunky oven fries

❖ MAKES 3 BABY PORTIONS OF GOUJONS

For the goujons:
175 g/6 oz skinless chicken breast
30 ml/2 tbsp plain (all-purpose) flour
A pinch of dried thyme (optional)
1 egg, beaten
50 g/2 oz/1 cup fresh white breadcrumbs
For the chunky oven fries:
100 g/4 oz potatoes, cut into fingers
15 ml/1 tbsp sunflower oil
To serve:
Baked beans in tomato sauce or peas

1. Cut the chicken breast into strips about 4 cm/1½ in long. Mix together the flour and thyme, if using. Dip the chicken strips in the flour, then in the beaten egg and finally in the breadcrumbs. Place a third of the goujons on a lightly greased baking (cookie) sheet.

2. Bring a pan of water to the boil, add the potato fingers and simmer for 3 minutes. Drain well.

3. Return the potato fingers to the pan and drizzle over the oil. Toss until lightly coated. Place in a single layer on the baking sheet, next to the goujons.

4. Bake on the top shelf of a preheated oven at 200°C/400°F/gas 6/fan oven 180°C for 15 minutes, turning the chicken and chips (fries) once, or until the chicken is cooked through and the chips are crisp and golden.

5. Transfer to a plate and allow to cool slightly before serving with baked beans or peas.

6. Divide the uncooked goujons into two portions. Open-freeze until solid, then put in freezerproof containers or bags and freeze until required. Alternatively, cover and store in the fridge for up to 24 hours.

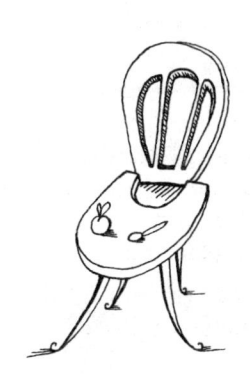

Mini meatballs in rich tomato sauce

❄ MAKES 2 ADULT PLUS 2 BABY PORTIONS

350 g/12 oz lean minced (ground) beef
50 g/2 oz/1 cup fresh white breadcrumbs
1 egg yolk
15 ml/1 tbsp chopped fresh parsley
Salt and freshly ground black pepper
15 ml/1 tbsp olive oil
1 medium onion, finely chopped
1 garlic clove, crushed
400 g/14 oz/1 large can of chopped tomatoes
2.5 ml/½ tsp dried mixed herbs
To serve:
Pasta or rice

1 Mix together the beef, breadcrumbs, egg yolk and parsley. Season with a little salt and pepper. With dampened hands, shape the mixture into 12 small balls.

2. Heat the oil in a frying pan (skillet), add the meatballs and cook over a medium heat for 5 minutes, turning frequently, until browned all over. Remove from the pan with a slotted spoon and set aside.

3. Add the onion and garlic to the pan and gently cook for 10 minutes until soft. Stir in the tomatoes and dried herbs and season with a little salt and pepper. Bring to the boil, cover and simmer for 10 minutes.

4. Place the meatballs in the sauce. Cover and simmer for a further 15 minutes or until cooked through.

5. Spoon a little of the sauce into a bowl and top with two meatballs. Allow to cool slightly before serving.

6. Remove a second baby portion, cool and freeze, or cover and store in the fridge for up to 24 hours.

7. Divide the remaining sauce and meatballs between the adults and serve with pasta or rice.

Tip
If preferred, the recipe can be divided into six baby portions.

Simple sweet and sour chicken

❋ MAKES 2 ADULT PLUS 1 BABY PORTION

15 ml/1 tbsp sunflower oil
2 skinless chicken breasts, cubed
10 ml/2 tsp cornflour (cornstarch)
10 ml/2 tsp sherry or white wine vinegar
10 ml/2 tsp light soy sauce
250 g/9 oz/1 small can of crushed pineapple
15 ml/1 tbsp tomato ketchup (catsup)
5 ml/1 tsp clear honey
1 medium carrot, diced
175 g/6 oz broccoli, cut into tiny florets
Salt and freshly ground black pepper
To serve:
Plain boiled rice or noodles

1 Heat the oil in a frying pan (skillet) and gently fry (sauté) the chicken for 5 minutes or until lightly browned. Remove from the pan and set aside.

2 Blend the cornflour with the sherry or vinegar and soy sauce. Add to the pan with the pineapple, ketchup and honey. Bring to the boil, stirring until thickened. Add the carrot and broccoli and simmer for 3 minutes.

3. Return the chicken and any juices to the pan and simmer for a further 4–5 minutes or until the vegetables are tender and the chicken cooked through.

4. Spoon a baby portion into a bowl and chop up the chicken into tiny pieces. Stir in a spoonful of rice or chopped noodles and leave to cool to the desired temperature before serving.

5. Season the remaining sweet and sour chicken with salt and pepper. Spoon on to a bed of rice or noodles and serve straight away.

Tip
If preferred, halve the recipe quantity, divide into five baby portions and freeze, or cover and store in the fridge for up to 24 hours.

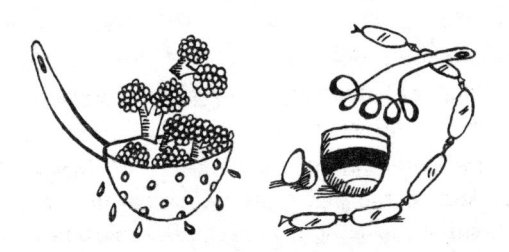

Special fried rice

MAKES 2 ADULT PLUS 1 BABY PORTION

225 g/8 oz/1 cup long-grain rice
5 ml/1 tsp sesame oil
30 ml/2 tbsp sunflower oil
6 spring onions (scallions), thinly sliced
1 medium carrot, coarsely grated
100 g/4 oz/2 cups beansprouts
50 g /2 oz frozen peas
100 g/4 oz small cooked peeled prawns (shrimp)
15 ml/1 tbsp light soy sauce
To serve:
Chilli sauce (optional)

1. Cook the rice in lightly salted boiling water for 8 minutes or until just tender. Drain well, rinse with boiling water, then drain again. Set aside.

2. Heat the oils in a wok or large frying pan (skillet). Add the spring onions and carrot and stir-fry for 2 minutes. Add the beansprouts and peas and stir-fry for 1 further minute.

3. Add the rice, prawns and soy sauce. Stir-fry for a further 3 minutes or until the rice and prawns are heated through.

From Baby to Toddler

4 Spoon a baby-sized portion into a bowl and allow to cool slightly before serving.

5 Divide the remainder between the adults and serve sprinkled with a little chilli sauce, if liked.

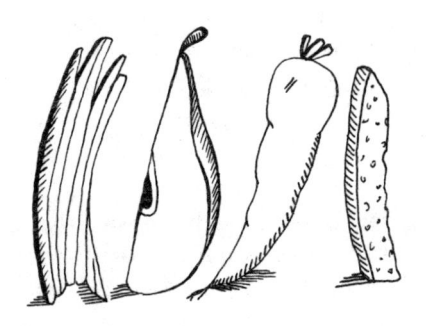

Sausage balls

Do read the section on allergies on page 21 before giving sesame seeds to your baby.

❇ MAKES 4 BABY PORTIONS

1 spring onion (scallion), finely chopped
225 g/8 oz good-quality sausagemeat
5 ml/1 tsp Worcestershire sauce
5 ml/1 tsp tomato purée (paste)
10 ml/2 tsp plain (all-purpose) flour
30 ml/2 tbsp sesame seeds
30 ml/2 tbsp sunflower oil

To serve:

Mashed potatoes and baked beans in tomato sauce or peas

1. Put the spring onion in a bowl with the sausagemeat, Worcestershire sauce and tomato purée and mix together well. Shape the mixture into 20 bite-sized balls.

2. Mix the flour and sesame seeds together in a small bowl. Roll the sausage balls in the seed mixture a few at a time until coated.

3 Heat the oil in a frying pan (skillet) and fry (sauté) five of the sausage balls for 5–6 minutes, turning frequently, until browned all over. Serve warm with mashed potatoes and baked beans or peas, or cold as finger food.

4 Open-freeze the remaining sausage balls until solid, then divide into portions, pack in freezerproof bags or containers and freeze until required.

Tip
When using the frozen portions, separate the sausage balls while still frozen and allow to defrost on a plate before cooking.

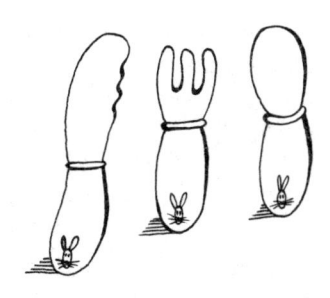

Toddler tuna tagliatelle

MAKES 2 ADULT PLUS 1 BABY PORTION

30 ml/2 tbsp olive oil
1 small onion, finely chopped
1 celery stick, finely chopped
1 garlic clove, crushed
200 g/7 oz/1 small can of chopped tomatoes
100 ml/3½ fl oz/scant ½ cup vegetable stock (see page 54)
1 bay leaf
200 g/7 oz/1 small can of tuna in oil
200 g/7 oz tagliatelle
15 g/½ oz/1 tbsp butter or margarine
15 ml/1 tbsp snipped fresh chives
Salt and freshly ground black pepper
To serve:
Finely grated Parmesan cheese (optional)

1. Heat the oil in a small saucepan and gently cook the onion and celery for 5 minutes. Add the garlic and cook for a further 5 minutes until soft.

2. Stir in the tomatoes, stock and bay leaf. Bring to the boil, then turn down the heat. Part-cover with a lid and simmer for 20 minutes.

3. Drain the tuna and flake. Remove the bay leaf from the sauce and stir in the tuna. Heat through for 1–2 minutes.

4. Meanwhile, cook the tagliatelle in lightly salted boiling water for 10 minutes, or according to the packet instructions. Drain thoroughly and toss in the butter or margarine and chives.

5. Spoon a little tagliatelle into a bowl and cut into small pieces. Top with a little of the sauce and allow to cool slightly before serving.

6. Season the remaining sauce with salt and freshly ground black pepper and serve to the adults with the tagliatelle. Sprinkle with Parmesan cheese, if liked.

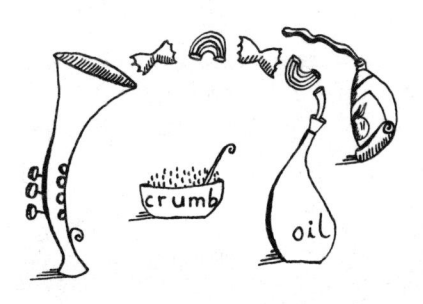

Plaice with carrot and orange sauce

MAKES 2 ADULT PLUS 1 BABY PORTION

5 small plaice fillets
300 ml/½ pint/1¼ cups vegetable stock (see page 54)
Salt and freshly ground black pepper
175 g/6 oz carrots, roughly chopped
Juice of ½ orange
1 bay leaf
2 sprigs of coriander (cilantro)
15 ml/1 tbsp cornflour (cornstarch)
60 ml/4 tbsp plain Greek yoghurt
15 ml/1 tbsp chopped fresh coriander

1. Skin the plaice fillets and rinse under cold water. Trim and roll up neatly, starting at the wider end and with the skinned side to the outside. Put in a lightly greased ovenproof dish. Spoon over 60 ml/4 tbsp of the stock, season lightly and cover with foil.

2. Put the carrots in a saucepan with the orange juice, the remaining stock, the bay leaf and sprigs of coriander. Bring to the boil, turn down the heat, cover and simmer for 20 minutes until tender.

3 Meanwhile, put the fish in a preheated oven at 190°C/375°F/gas 5/fan oven 170°C and bake for 15–20 minutes or until cooked.

4 Remove the bay leaf and coriander sprigs from the carrots, then purée until smooth. Rinse out the pan. Blend the cornflour and yoghurt together in the pan, then stir in the carrot purée. Reheat gently until thickened, stirring continuously.

5 Serve two plaice fillets for each adult and one for baby. Spoon over the carrot sauce and sprinkle with the chopped coriander.

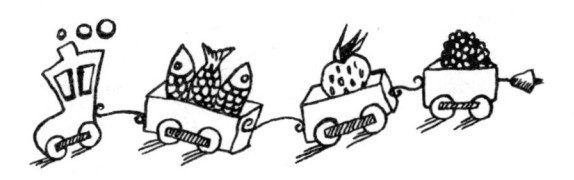

Special fish supper

MAKES 2 ADULT PLUS 1 BABY PORTION

350 g/12 oz new potatoes, scrubbed
25 g/1 oz/2 tbsp butter or margarine
25 g/1 oz/¼ cup plain (all-purpose) flour
250 ml/8 fl oz/1 cup milk
Smoked cod or haddock, skinned and boned
50 g/2 oz/½ cup finely grated Red Leicester cheese
Freshly ground black pepper

1. Cook the potatoes in boiling salted water for 15 minutes. Drain and leave until cool enough to handle, then slice.

2. Put the butter or margarine, flour and milk in a saucepan and slowly bring to the boil, stirring all the time, until smooth and thickened.

3. Cut the fish into small cubes and stir into the sauce. Simmer for 4–5 minutes until the fish is cooked. Remove from the heat and stir in three-quarters of the cheese.

4. Spoon a little of the fish mixture into a greased 150 ml/ ¼ pint/⅔ cup ramekin (custard cup). Season the remainder with pepper and spoon into a 750 ml/1¼ pint/3 cup shallow flameproof dish.

5 Lay the potato slices over the fish in both dishes and sprinkle with the remaining cheese. Place under a medium grill (broiler) for 4–5 minutes until the potatoes and cheese are golden brown and bubbling. Cool the baby portion to the desired temperature before serving.

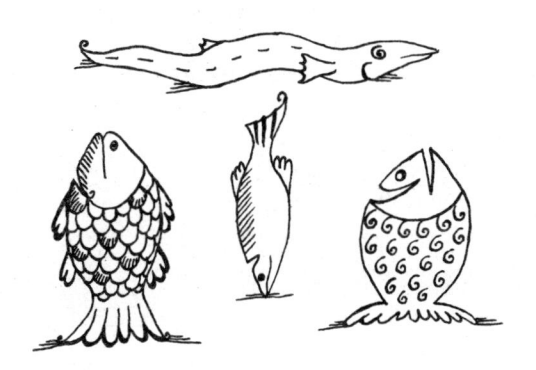

Cod creole

Creole is a delicious Caribbean style of cooking in which the food is prepared with peppers, tomatoes and rice. The usual dash of hot and spicy Tabasco sauce has been left out of this recipe!

❋ MAKES 3 BABY PORTIONS

300 ml/½ pint/1¼ cups vegetable stock (see page 54)
5 ml/1 tsp tomato purée (paste)
½ red (bell) pepper, seeded and finely chopped
50 g/2 oz/¼ cup long-grain rice
100 g/4 oz skinless cod

1 Pour the stock into a small saucepan, add the tomato purée and bring to the boil. Add the pepper, rice and fish, then turn down the heat.

2 Part-cover the pan with a lid, then simmer gently for 15 minutes or until the rice and fish are cooked.

3 Lift out the fish with a slotted spoon and flake, discarding any bones. Stir the flaked fish back into the rice mixture and spoon a third into a bowl. Allow to cool slightly, if necessary, before serving.

4 Divide the rest of the mixture into portions, cover and freeze, or store in the fridge for up to 24 hours.

Fluffy cheese on toast

MAKES 1 LARGE BABY PORTION

15 g/½ oz/1 tbsp butter or margarine
10 ml/2 tsp plain (all-purpose) flour
75 ml/5 tbsp milk
25 g/1 oz/¼ cup finely grated Cheddar cheese
1 egg, separated
2 slices of toast

1. Melt the butter or margarine in a small saucepan over a gentle heat. Stir in the flour and cook for a few seconds. Add the milk, a little at a time. Simmer for 1 minute until thickened, then remove from the heat.

2. Stir in the cheese until melted, then the egg yolk. Whisk the egg white until stiff and fold into the mixture.

3. Spoon the mixture on top of the toast and cook under a low grill (broiler) for 4–5 minutes until cooked through, golden brown and puffy. Cool for a few minutes before serving.

Egg in a basket

MAKES 1 BABY PORTION

1 slice of white or wholemeal bread
15 g/½ oz/1 tbsp butter or margarine
1 egg
15 ml/1 tbsp milk

1. Remove the crusts from the bread and thinly spread both sides with most of the butter or margarine. Press the bread into a patty tin (pan) to form a basket. Bake in a preheated oven at 200°C/400°F/gas 6/fan oven 180°C for 8 minutes or until lightly browned.

2. Meanwhile, melt the remaining butter or margarine in a small pan. Whisk together the egg and milk and pour into the pan. Cook over a gentle heat, stirring all the time until lightly set.

3. Place the bread basket on a plate and spoon in the scrambled egg. Serve straight away.

Tip
Flavour the scrambled egg by stirring in a skinned, seeded and diced tomato or a chopped thin slice of ham.

Bacon and tomato scramble

MAKES 1 BABY PORTION

1 rasher (slice) of streaky bacon, rinded
1 ripe tomato
1 egg
15 ml/1 tbsp milk
15 g/½ oz/1 tbsp butter or margarine
To serve:
Fingers of hot buttered toast

1. Chop the bacon into small pieces. Dry-fry in a small non-stick frying pan (skillet) for 3–4 minutes until crisp. Remove and set aside.

2. Meanwhile, plunge the tomato into boiling water for 1 minute. Remove, then peel, halve and remove the seeds. Finely chop the flesh.

3. Beat the egg with the milk. Melt the butter or margarine in the frying pan over a low heat, then add the egg mixture and chopped tomato. Cook slowly, stirring all the time, until thickened and set. Spoon on to a plate.

4. Sprinkle over the bacon pieces and allow to cool for a minute or two. Serve with fingers of buttered toast.

Mini toad-in-the-hole

If you don't have a Yorkshire pudding tin (pan) with four 10 cm/4 in compartments, use a bun tin to make eight small Yorkshire puddings and cook for slightly less time.

MAKES **4** BABY PORTIONS

225 g/8 oz sausages
15 g/½ oz/1 tbsp white vegetable fat (shortening)
100 g/4 oz mixed vegetables, such as carrots, broccoli or courgettes (zucchini), cut into bite-sized chunks
50 g/2 oz/½ cup plain (all-purpose) flour
A pinch of salt
1 egg
175 ml/6 fl oz/¾ cup milk

1. Cut the sausages into 3 cm/1¼ in slices. Use the fat to lightly grease the compartments of a four-hole Yorkshire pudding tin, then divide the sausage slices between them.

2. Cook the vegetables in boiling water or steam for 2–3 minutes until almost tender. Drain well.

3. Put the Yorkshire pudding tin in a preheated oven at 220°C/425°F/gas 7/fan oven 200°C for 5 minutes. This will heat the tin and start cooking the sausages.

4. Meanwhile, sift the flour and salt into a bowl and make a well in the centre. Break the egg into the well, then pour in half the milk. Gradually mix the flour into the liquid to make a smooth batter, then whisk in the remaining milk.

5. Divide the vegetables between the compartments of the tin and pour over the batter. Bake on the top shelf in the oven for 30 minutes or until well risen and golden brown.

6. Remove from the tin and allow to cool for a few minutes before serving. Children may find them easier to eat with their fingers, rather than a knife and fork.

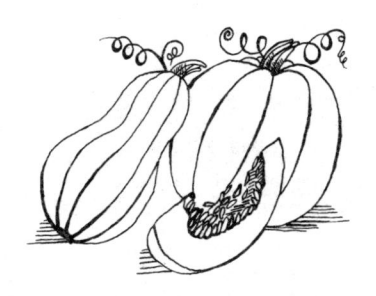

Squeakies

These mini 'bubble and squeak' fritters may be served as finger food or as part of a meal.

MAKES 1 BABY PORTION

100 g/4 oz potato, coarsely grated
50 g/2 oz cooked cabbage, finely chopped
15 ml/1 tbsp frozen peas, defrosted
30 ml/2 tbsp plain (all-purpose) flour
1 egg
30 ml/2 tbsp sunflower oil

1. Squeeze any excess liquid out of the potato, then pat dry on kitchen paper (paper towels).
2. Add the cabbage and peas to the grated potato. Sprinkle over the flour and mix together. Add the egg and mix again.
3. Heat the oil in a frying pan (skillet) and drop in tablespoonfuls of the mixture. Flatten with the back of a fork and cook for 4–5 minutes on each side until crisp and golden.
4. Drain on kitchen paper and allow to cool slightly before serving.

Strawberry wobble

Most children enjoy jelly, so try turning it into a nutritious dessert with the addition of evaporated milk.

MAKES 2 BABY PORTIONS

½ packet of strawberry jelly (jello)
120 ml/4 fl oz/½ cup boiling water
175 g/6 oz/1 small can of evaporated milk

To decorate:
A few fresh strawberries, hulled and quartered (optional)

1. Cut the jelly into small cubes. Pour the boiling water over and stir until the jelly has dissolved. Leave to cool for 10 minutes.

2. Stir in the evaporated milk, then pour into two small bowls or jelly moulds. Leave to cool completely, then transfer to the fridge and chill until set.

3. Serve in the bowl or dip one of the moulds briefly into very hot water and turn out on to a plate to serve. Decorate with a few fresh strawberries, if liked.

4. Store the remaining portion in the fridge for up to 24 hours.

From Baby to Toddler

Baked maple apples

Although cooking (tart) apples are traditionally used for baking, eating (dessert) apples are much sweeter and a better size for a toddler to tackle.

MAKES 2 BABY PORTIONS

30 ml/2 tbsp raisins
75 ml/5 tbsp apple juice or water
2 small eating (dessert) apples
15 g/½ oz/1 tbsp butter or margarine, softened
30 ml/2 tbsp maple syrup
A small pinch of ground cinnamon

To serve:
Ice cream

1. Put the raisins in a small bowl with the apple juice or water and leave to soak for at least 20 minutes.

2. Core the apples and prick the skins with a fork or skewer in several places to prevent them from bursting. Put the apples in a small, shallow ovenproof dish.

3. Mix the butter or margarine, maple syrup and cinnamon together. Remove the raisins from the apple juice and stir into the mixture. Spoon into the centre of each apple. Pour the remaining soaking liquid into the dish.

4. Cover the apples with a piece of greased foil and bake in a preheated oven at 180°C/350°F/gas 4/fan oven 160°C for 40 minutes or until the apples are very tender.

5. Scoop the pulp from one of the apples into a bowl and allow to cool slightly before serving with ice cream.

6. Allow the remaining apple to cool. Cover and keep in the fridge for up to 24 hours.

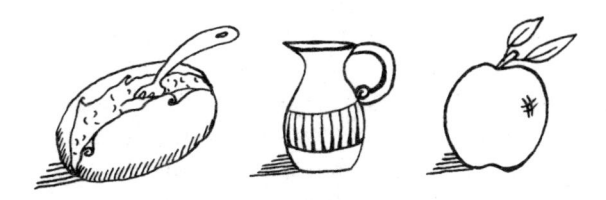

Rich chocolate pudding

During cooking, this delicious dessert separates into two layers; a thick chocolate sauce at the bottom, topped with a fudgy sponge.

MAKES 2 ADULT PLUS 1 BABY PORTION

For the sponge:
50 g/2 oz/¼ cup butter or margarine
50 g/2 oz/¼ cup caster (superfine) sugar
1 egg, beaten
40 g/1½ oz/⅓ cup self-raising (self-rising) flour
15 g/½ oz/2 tbsp cocoa (unsweetened chocolate) powder
2.5 ml/½ tsp baking powder
1.5 ml/¼ tsp vanilla essence (extract)
15 ml/1 tbsp milk
For the sauce:
40 g/1½ oz/3 tbsp light muscovado sugar
15 g/½ oz/1 tbsp cocoa powder
120 ml/4 fl oz/½ cup cold water

1 Make the sponge. Cream the butter or margarine and sugar together until light and fluffy. Gradually add the egg, beating well after each addition. Sift the flour, cocoa powder and baking powder over the mixture. Add the vanilla essence to the milk and gently fold in.

2. Spoon the mixture into a well greased 600 ml/1 pint/2½ cup ovenproof dish and level the top with the back of a spoon.

3. Make the sauce. Mix the muscovado sugar and cocoa powder together and sprinkle over the sponge mixture. Carefully pour over the cold water.

4. Bake in a preheated oven at 190°C/375°F/gas 5/fan oven 170°C for 30–35 minutes or until the pudding has risen and is firm to the touch.

5. Spoon the baby portion of sponge and sauce into a bowl and allow to cool slightly before serving.

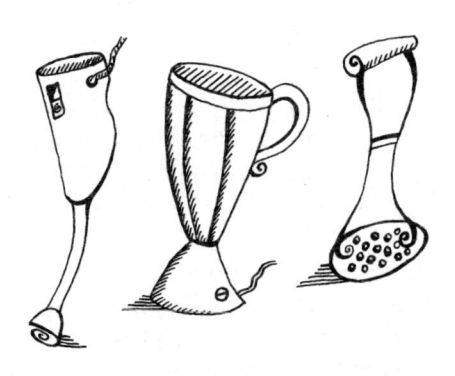

Home-made ice cream

❇ MAKES 8 BABY PORTIONS

300 ml/½ pint/1¼ cups milk
3 egg yolks
50 g/2 oz/¼ cup caster (superfine) sugar
2.5 ml/½ tsp cornflour (cornstarch)
2.5 ml/½ tsp vanilla essence (extract)
300 ml/½ pint/1¼ cups whipping cream

1 Pour the milk into a saucepan and heat to boiling point. Meanwhile, whisk the egg yolks, sugar, cornflour and vanilla essence together in a bowl until thick and creamy. Gradually whisk in the hot milk, then pour back into the pan.

2 Cook the custard over a low heat, stirring all the time, until thick enough to coat the back of a wooden spoon. Do not allow to boil. Pour into a bowl, cover with a piece of dampened greaseproof (waxed) paper to prevent a skin forming and leave to cool.

3 Whisk the cream until just thick, then fold it into the cold custard. Pour into a shallow container and freeze, whisking two or three times during freezing to break down the ice crystals. Alternatively, churn in an ice cream maker.

4. Scoop the ice cream into bowls and allow to soften slightly at room temperature before serving.

Tip:
Ice cream that has softened should never be refrozen, or you could risk food poisoning.

Strawberry ice cream

Blend 225 g/8 oz of strawberries to a purée in a food processor with 45 ml/3 tbsp of icing (confectioners') sugar. Rub through a sieve (strainer) to remove the pips, then stir into the cold custard before folding in the whipped cream.

Chocolate ice cream

Stir 75 g/3 oz of milk chocolate drops into the hot custard before transferring to a bowl to cool.

Iced raspberry and banana yoghurt

❋ MAKES 6 BABY PORTIONS

225 g/8 oz raspberries
1 medium ripe banana
25 g/1 oz/2 tbsp soft light brown sugar
150 ml/¼ pint/⅔ cup plain Greek yoghurt

1. Reserve a few raspberries for decorating, then put the rest in a food processor with the banana and sugar and purée until smooth. Press through a sieve (strainer) to remove the pips.

2. Stir the yoghurt into the fruit purée. Pour into a shallow container and freeze, whisking two or three times during freezing to break up the ice crystals. Alternatively, churn in an ice cream maker.

3. Scoop into bowls and allow to soften slightly at room temperature before serving decorated with a few fresh raspberries.

Cheese cookies

❋ MAKES 12

75 g/3 oz/¾ cup self-raising (self-rising) flour
25 g/1 oz/¼ cup plain (all-purpose) wholemeal flour
50 g/2 oz/⅓ cup ground rice
A pinch of salt
100 g/4 oz/½ cup soft margarine
50 g/2 oz/½ cup finely grated Cheddar cheese

1. Put all the ingredients in a mixing bowl and stir together with a wooden spoon until combined. Knead on a lightly floured work surface for a few seconds until smooth, then shape into a roll about 15 cm/6 in long. Wrap in clingfilm (plastic wrap) and chill in the fridge for 1 hour.

2. Cut the roll into slices 1 cm/½ in thick and place on a lightly greased baking (cookie) sheet. Bake in a preheated oven at 190°C/375°F/gas 5/fan oven 170°C for 12–15 minutes or until lightly browned.

3. Leave to cool on the baking sheet for 5 minutes, then transfer to a wire cooling rack. When cold, store in an airtight tin for up to a week, or pack into a freezerproof bag or container and freeze until required.

Banana cake with fudge frosting

MAKES 9 SQUARES

For the cake:
100 g/4 oz/1 cup plain (all-purpose) flour
2.5 ml/½ tsp baking powder
2.5 ml/½ tsp bicarbonate of soda (baking soda)
1 egg
15 ml/1 tbsp golden (light corn) syrup
100 ml/3½ fl oz/scant ½ cup milk
60 ml/4 tbsp sunflower oil
1 ripe banana, mashed

For the fudge frosting:
25 g/1 oz/2 tbsp butter or margarine
10 ml/2 tsp milk
1.5 ml/¼ tsp vanilla essence (extract)
15 ml/1 tbsp cocoa (unsweetened chocolate) powder
175 g/6 oz/1 cup icing (confectioners') sugar

1 Make the cake. Grease and line an 18 cm/7 in square tin (pan) with greaseproof (waxed) paper. Sift the flour, baking powder and bicarbonate of soda into a mixing bowl.

2. Beat the egg, golden syrup, milk, oil and banana together. Make a well in the middle of the dry ingredients and pour in the banana mixture. Beat together until mixed, then pour into the prepared tin.

3. Bake on the middle shelf of a preheated oven at 160°C/325°F/gas 3/fan oven 145°C for 25 minutes or until springy to the touch. Turn out on to a wire rack and leave to cool.

4. Make the frosting. Gently heat the butter or margarine, milk and vanilla essence together in a small pan until melted. Sift the cocoa powder and icing sugar into a bowl and stir in the warm melted butter or margarine mixture. Beat together until light and fluffy.

5. Spread the frosting over the top of the cake. Cut into squares to serve. Store in an airtight container for up to 3 days.

Yoghurt and raisin muffins

❋ MAKES 12

50 g/2 oz/⅓ cup raisins
45 ml/3 tbsp orange juice
225 g/8 oz/2 cups plain (all-purpose) flour
7.5 ml/1½ tsp baking powder
5 ml/1 tsp bicarbonate of soda (baking soda)
2.5 ml/½ tsp ground cinnamon
A pinch of salt
50 g/2 oz/¼ cup light soft brown sugar
50 g/2 oz/½ cup fine oatmeal
1 egg
120 ml/4 fl oz/½ cup milk
250 ml/8 fl oz/1 cup plain Greek yoghurt
40 g/1½ oz/3 tbsp butter or margarine, melted and cooled

1. Put the raisins in a small bowl, spoon over the orange juice and leave to soak for 1 hour. Line a 12-section muffin tin (pan) with paper muffin cases.

2. Sift the flour, baking powder, bicarbonate of soda, cinnamon and salt into a mixing bowl. Stir in the sugar and oatmeal. Make a well in the middle.

3. Beat the egg with the milk. Stir in the raisins and orange juice, the yoghurt and butter or margarine. Add to the dry ingredients and stir briefly until just mixed.

4. Divide the mixture equally between the muffin cases. Bake in a preheated oven at 200°C/400°F/gas 6/fan oven 180°C for 20 minutes until well risen and firm.

5. Cool the muffins on a wire rack. Remove the paper cases before serving warm or cold. Store in an airtight tin for up to 3 days, or pack into a freezerproof container and freeze.

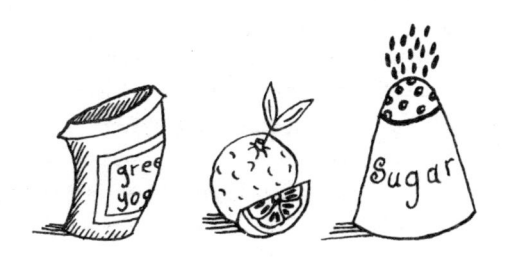

From Baby to Toddler

Iced carrot cake

See the information on allergies on page 21 before using ground almonds for your baby.

❋ MAKES 9 SQUARES

For the cake:
100 g/4 oz/½ cup butter or margarine, softened
100 g/4 oz/½ cup soft light brown sugar
2 eggs, beaten
75 g/3 oz/¾ cup self-raising (self-rising) flour
2.5 ml/½ tsp baking powder
1.5 ml/¼ tsp mixed (apple-pie) spice
15 ml/1 tbsp milk
25 g/1 oz/¼ cup ground almonds
150 g/5 oz carrots, coarsely grated
For the icing (frosting):
150 g/5 oz Mascarpone cheese
15 ml/1 tbsp orange juice
15 ml/1 tbsp icing (confectioners') sugar, sifted

1 Make the cake. Grease and line an 18 cm/7 in square tin (pan). Cream the butter or margarine and sugar until pale and fluffy. Add the eggs a little at a time, beating well after each addition.

2 Sift the flour, baking powder and mixed spice over the mixture and fold in with the milk and ground almonds. Finally, fold in the grated carrot.

3 Turn the mixture into the prepared tin and level the top with the back of a spoon. Bake in a preheated oven at 180°C/350°F/gas 4/fan oven 160°C for 35 minutes or until well risen and firm. Leave in the tin for 5 minutes, then turn out on to a wire rack to cool.

4 Make the icing. Beat the Mascarpone, orange juice and icing sugar together until smooth. Spread over the top of the cake. Cut the cake into squares and store in the fridge until ready to serve, or open-freeze, then wrap individual portions in clingfilm (plastic wrap) and freeze until required.

Index

allergies and food intolerance 21–2
apple
  apple purée 30
  apple and raspberry purée 49
  apple and raspberry ripple yoghurt 86
  baked maple apples 172–3
  baked sweet potato and apple 83
  cream of fruit purée 32
  creamed rice with apple or pear 47
  finger food 94
  orchard fruit fool 90
  savoury pork and apple casserole 68–9
  two-fruit purée 32
apricot
  apricot fool 131
  apricot smoothie 50
autumn vegetable trio 40

baby rice
  apricot smoothie 50
  cream of carrot and courgette 73
  cream of pumpkin 46
  how to make up 29
bacon
  bacon and bean feast 102–3
  bacon and tomato scramble 167
baked beans
  bacon and bean feast 102–3
  beefy bean dinner 98
  paprika pork with rice and beans 106
baked egg custard 89
baked maple apples 172–3
baked sweet potato and apple 83
banana
  banana cake with fudge frosting 180–1
  banana cream 88
  banana and kiwi fruit 48
  banana purée 30
  finger food 94
  iced raspberry and banana yoghurt 178
  steamed banana custard 130
  two-fruit purée 32
beansprouts
  special fried rice 154–5
beef
  beef and carrot braise 66–7
  beefy bean dinner 98
  chunky beef casserole 96–7
  mini meatballs in rich tomato sauce 150–1
blackberries
  blushing pear dessert 87
blushing fruit salad 52
blushing pear dessert 87
bread
  egg in a basket 166
  finger food 94
  fluffy cheese on toast 165
  French toast fingers 124
  teething rusks 92
breakfast at 5–6 months
  apple and raspberry purée 49
  apricot smoothie 50
  banana and kiwi fruit 48
  blushing fruit salad 52
  cream of plum and pear 51
  creamed rice with apple or pear 47
  vanilla peach purée 53
  see also lunch at 5–6 months
breakfast cereal, finger food 94
broccoli
  broccoli and cauliflower cheese 64–5
  cheesy cod and broccoli 112
  country pork with broccoli 99
butter baked salmon with dill 113
butternut squash purée 34

cabbage
  squeakies 170

Index

cake
  banana cake with fudge frosting 180–1
  iced carrot cake 184–5
carrot
  autumn vegetable trio 40
  beef and carrot braise 66–7
  butter baked salmon with dill 113
  carrot purée 33
  chicken casserole 41
  chicken with garden vegetables 62
  chicken and vegetable bites 109
  cream of carrot and courgette 73
  creamy carrot and coriander with lentils 74
  creamy carrot mousse 114–5
  finger food 94
  fisherman's pie 110–11
  iced carrot cake 184–5
  plaice with carrot and orange sauce 160–1
casseroles
  beef and carrot braise 66–7
  chicken casserole 41
  chunky beef 96–7
  crumble-topped lamb 140–1
  savoury pork and apple 68–9
cauliflower, broccoli and cauliflower cheese 64–5
celeriac (celery root)
  creamed potato and celeriac with cheese 72–3
celery
  finger food 94
celery root *see* celeriac
cheese
  bacon and bean feast 102–3
  broccoli and cauliflower cheese 64–5
  cheese cookies 179
  cheesy cod and broccoli 112
  cream cheese and ham pasta 123
  creamed potato and celeriac with cheese 72–3
  easy cheese and tomato pizza puffs 136–7
  finger food 94
  fluffy cheese on toast 165

chicken
  chicken casserole 41
  chicken with garden vegetables 62
  chicken goujons with chunky oven fries 148–9
  chicken satay sticks 142–3
  chicken and vegetable bites 109
  creamy chicken korma 138–9
  crunchy chicken nuggets 135
  finger food 94
  main meal minestrone 118–9
  one-pot chicken and rice 63
  simple sweet and sour chicken 152–3
chips (fries)
  chunky oven fries 148–9
chocolate
  chocolate drop pudding 125
  chocolate ice cream 177
  chocolate milk jelly 128–9
  chocolate rice pudding 82
  rich chocolate pudding 174–5
cod
  cheesy cod and broccoli 112
  cod and courgette savoury 42–3
  cod creole 164
  creamed cod and corn chowder 61
  fisherman's pie 110–11
  quick fish kedgeree 75
  special fish supper 162–3
commercially prepared food 20
cookies
  cheese 179
corn *see* sweetcorn
country pork with broccoli 99
courgette (zucchini)
  cod and courgette savoury 42–3
  cream of carrot and courgette 73
  Mediterranean vegetables with pasta 80–1
couscous
  fruity lamb couscous 104–5
cream of carrot and courgette 73
cream cheese and ham pasta 123
cream of fruit purée 32
cream of plum and pear 51

187

Index

cream of pumpkin 46
creamed cod and corn chowder 61
creamed potato and celeriac with cheese 72–3
creamed rice with apple or pear 47
creamy carrot and coriander with lentils 74
creamy carrot mousse 114–5
creamy chicken korma 138–9
crumble-topped lamb casserole 140–1
crunchy fish fingers 146–7
curry
  creamy chicken korma 138–9
custard
  orchard fruit fool 90
  pear and prune 84–5

defrosting baby food 15
dill
  butter baked salmon with dill 113
drinks
  fruit juice 19–20
  importance of milk 7, 8–9

easy cheese and tomato pizza puffs 136–7
egg
  bacon and tomato scramble 167
  baked egg custard 89
  egg in a basket 166
  fluffy cheese on toast 165
  French toast fingers 124
  home-made ice cream 176–7
  vanilla creams 126

finger foods 94
fish
  butter baked salmon with dill 113
  cheesy cod and broccoli 112
  cod and courgette savoury 42–3
  cod creole 164
  creamed cod and corn chowder 61
  crunchy fish fingers 146–7
  fisherman's pie 110–11
  plaice with carrot and orange sauce 160–1
  poached fish with pea and potato purée 70–1
  quick fish kedgeree 75
  special fish supper 162–3
  toddler tuna tagliatelle 158–9
  see also types of fish
fisherman's pie 110–11
flaked rice
  chocolate rice pudding 82
  creamed rice with apple or pear 47
fluffy cheese on toast 165
food
  approximate ages for introducing 16–8
  nutritional value 6–7
  hygiene 13–14
  intolerance 21–2
  seasoning 93
  sugar content 19
  to avoid
    at 4 months 26
    at 5 months 36
    at 6–9 months 59
    at 6–12 months 95
  see also solid food
freezing baby food 14, 15
French (green) beans
  chicken with garden vegetables 62
French toast fingers 124
fromage frais
  blushing pear dessert 87
  fruit and fromage frais jelly 127
  potato and watercress purée with fromage frais 78
fruit
  blushing fruit salad 52
  cream of fruit purée 32
  fresh fruity jelly 127
  fruit and fromage frais jelly 127
  fruity lamb couscous 104–5
  orchard fruit fool 90
  two-fruit purée 32
fruity lamb couscous 104–5
fussy eaters 133–4

188

Index

gluten intolerance 22
green (French) beans
  chicken with garden vegetables 62

haddock
  fisherman's pie 110–11
  special fish supper 162–3
ham
  cream cheese and ham pasta 123
  spaghetti junction 121
honey
  as food to avoid 17, 20, 26, 36, 59, 95

ice cream
  chocolate 177
  home-made 176–7
  strawberry 177
iced carrot cake 184–5
iced raspberry and banana yoghurt 178
iron in diet 6–7

jelly
  chocolate milk 128–9
  fresh fruity 127
  fruit and fromage frais 127
  strawberry wobble 171

kiwi
  banana and kiwi fruit 48

lactose intolerance 22
lamb
  crumble-topped lamb casserole 140–1
  fruity lamb couscous 104–5
  lamb and lentil lasagne 144–5
  lamb and lentil supper 107
  shepherds' pie 100–1
leek and potato purée 76–7
lentils *see* red lentils
lumpy food, introducing 56
lunch at 5–6 months
  autumn vegetable trio 40
  chicken casserole 41
  cod and courgette savoury 42–3
  cream of pumpkin 46
  meal planner 37–8
  red lentils with vegetables 39
  sweet potato and spinach 44
  turkey with peas and sweetcorn 45

macaroni
  beefy bean dinner 98
main meal minestrone 118–9
meal planning
  4–5 months 27–8
  5–6 months 37–8
  making meal times easy 22–3
meatballs in rich tomato sauce, mini 150–1
Mediterranean vegetables with pasta 80–1
melon, blushing fruit salad 52
microwave cooking and reheating 15, 29
milk
  in cooking 14, 56
  importance of hygiene 7, 8–9, 14, 18–9
minced meat
  beefy bean dinner 98
  lamb and lentil lasagne 144–5
  mini meatballs in rich tomato
    sauce 150–1
  shepherds' pie 100–1
mixed vegetable risotto 60
muffins
  yoghurt and raisin muffins 182–3
mushrooms
  pasta with mushroom sauce 116–7

nectarine
  vanilla peach purée 53
nuts 17, 18, 20

one-pot chicken and rice 63
orchard fruit fool 90–1

papaya (pawpaw)
  cream of fruit purée 32
  papaya purée 31
  two-fruit purée 32
parsnip purée 33

Index

pasta
  beefy bean dinner 98
  cream cheese and ham pasta 123
  finger food 94
  lamb and lentil lasagne 144–5
  main meal minestrone 118–9
  Mediterranean vegetables with pasta 80–1
  pasta with mushroom sauce 116–7
  pasta primavera 120
  spaghetti junction 121
  toddler tuna tagliatelle 158–9
pawpaw *see* papaya (pawpaw)
peach
  vanilla peach purée 53
peanut butter
  allergies 22
  chicken satay sticks 142–3
pear
  blushing fruit salad 52
  blushing pear dessert 87
  cream of fruit purée 32
  cream of plum and pear 51
  creamed rice with apple or pear 47
  finger food 94
  pear and prune custard 84–5
  pear purée 31
  two-fruit purée 32
peas
  poached fish with pea and potato purée 70–1
  squeakies 170
  turkey with peas and sweetcorn 45
peppers (bell peppers)
  cod creole 164
  Mediterranean vegetables with pasta 80–1
  mixed vegetable risotto 60
pineapple
  simple sweet and sour chicken 152–3
pizza
  easy cheese and tomato pizza puffs 136–7
plaice
  crunchy fish fingers 146–7
  plaice with carrot and orange sauce 160–1

poached fish with pea and potato purée 70–1
plum
  cream of plum and pear 51
  orchard fruit fool 90–1
poached fish with pea and potato purée 70–1
pork
  country pork with broccoli 99
  paprika pork with rice and beans 106
  savoury pork and apple casserole 68–9
potato
  autumn vegetable trio 40
  bacon and bean feast 102–3
  cheesy cod and broccoli 112
  chicken casserole 41
  chicken with garden vegetables 62
  chicken goujons with chunky oven fries 148–9
  chicken and vegetable bites 109
  creamed potato and celeriac with cheese 72–3
  fisherman's pie 110–11
  leek and potato purée 76–7
  poached fish with pea and potato purée 70–1
  potato purée 34
  potato and watercress purée with fromage frais 78
  shepherds' pie 100–1
  special fish supper 162–3
  squeakies 170
  turkey with peas and sweetcorn 45
  see also sweet potato
prawns (shrimp)
  special fried rice 154–5
prune
  pear and prune custard 84–5
puddings
  apple and raspberry ripple yoghurt 86
  apricot fool 131
  baked egg custard 89
  baked maple apples 172–3
  baked sweet potato and apple 83

Index

banana cream 88
blushing pear dessert 87
chocolate drop pudding 125
chocolate milk jelly 128–9
chocolate rice pudding 82
fresh fruity jelly 127
fruit and fromage frais jelly 127
home-made ice cream 176–7
iced raspberry and banana yoghurt 178
orchard fruit fool 90
pear and prune custard 84–5
rich chocolate pudding 174–5
steamed banana custard 130
strawberry wobble 171
vanilla creams 126
pumpkin
  cream of pumpkin 46
purées
  microwave cooking 29
  apple 30
  banana 30
  butternut squash 34
  carrot, swede or parsnip 33
  cream of fruit 32
  papaya 31
  pear 31
  potato 34
  two-fruit 32

quick fish kedgeree 75

raisins
  baked maple apples 172–3
  yoghurt and raisin muffins 182–3
raspberry
  apple and raspberry purée 49
  apple and raspberry ripple yoghurt 86
  blushing fruit salad 52
  blushing pear dessert 87
  iced raspberry and banana yoghurt 178
red lentils
  creamy carrot and coriander with lentils 74
  lamb and lentil lasagne 144–5
  lamb and lentil supper 107
  red lentils with vegetables 39
reheating baby food 15
rice
  chocolate drop pudding 125
  cod creole 164
  mixed vegetable risotto 60
  one-pot chicken and rice 63
  paprika pork with rice and beans 106
  quick fish kedgeree 75
  special fried rice 154–5
  turkey and tomato hotpot 108
  see also baby rice; flaked rice
rich chocolate pudding 174–5
rusks
  teething 92
rutabaga *see* swede (rutabaga)

salmon
  butter baked salmon with dill 113
salt 6
sandwiches, mini
  as finger food 94
sausagemeat
  sausage balls 156–7
sausages
  mini toad-in-the-hole 168–9
savoury pork and apple casserole 68–9
savoury spinach custard 122
self-feeding 57–8
shellfish 17, 22, 26, 36, 59, 95
shepherds' pie 100–1
shrimp (prawns)
  special fried rice 154–5
simple sweet and sour chicken 152–3
solid food
  equipment 11–13
  freezing 15
  getting started 8–9
  thawing 15
  weaning from milk feeds 7–8
  weaning tips 10
spaghetti junction 121
special fish supper 162–3

Index

special fried rice 154–5
spinach
  savoury spinach custard 122
  sweet potato and spinach 44
squeakies 170
steamed banana custard 130
stock
  home-made vegetable 54–5
strawberry
  blushing pear dessert 87
  ice cream 177
  strawberry wobble 171
swede (rutabaga)
  autumn vegetable trio 40
  swede purée 33
sweet potato
  baked sweet potato and apple 83
  creamed cod and corn chowder 61
  lamb and lentil supper 107
  sweet potato and spinach 44
sweetcorn (corn)
  chicken and vegetable bites 109
  creamed cod and corn chowder 61
  turkey with peas and sweetcorn 45

teething rusks 92
thawing baby food 15
toad-in-the-hole, mini 168–9
toddler tuna tagliatelle 158–9
tofu
  banana cream 88
tomato
  bacon and tomato scramble 167
  easy cheese and tomato pizza puffs 136–7
  Mediterranean vegetables with pasta 80–1
  mini meatballs in rich tomato sauce 150–1
  pasta with mushroom sauce 116–7
  toddler tuna tagliatelle 158–9
  turkey and tomato hotpot 108
tuna
  toddler tuna tagliatelle 158–9

turkey
  turkey with peas and sweetcorn 45
  turkey and tomato hotpot 108
vanilla
  home-made ice cream 176–7
  steamed banana custard 130
  vanilla creams 126
  vanilla peach purée 53
vegetables
  autumn vegetable trio 40
  chicken with garden vegetables 62
  chicken and vegetable bites 109
  crumble-topped lamb casserole 140–1
  home-made vegetable stock 54–5
  main meal minestrone 118–9
  Mediterranean vegetables with pasta 80–1
  mini toad-in-the-hole 168–9
  mixed vegetable risotto 60
  pasta primavera 120
  red lentils with vegetables 39
  simple sweet and sour chicken 152–3
  special fried rice 154–5
  spaghetti junction 121
  vegetable medley 79
  see also types of vegetables
vegetarian and vegan diets 20–1
vitamin drops 7

watercress
  potato and watercress purée with fromage frais 78
weaning 7–10
  see also food; solid food

yeast extract
  teething rusks 92
yoghurt
  apple and raspberry ripple yoghurt 86
  apricot fool 131
  creamy chicken korma 138–9
  iced raspberry and banana yoghurt 178
  yoghurt and raisin muffins 182–3